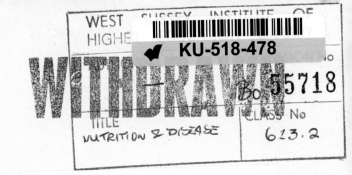

NUTRITION AND DISEASE

CROOM HELM APPLIED BIOLOGY SERIES

Edited by Peter Baron, BSc. Hons, PhD

Nutrition and Disease
Edited by R.J. Jarrett

NUTRITION AND DISEASE

Edited by R.J. Jarrett

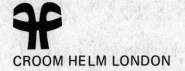

CROOM HELM LONDON

©1979 R.J. Jarrett
Croom Helm Ltd, 2-10 St John's Road, London SW11

British Library Cataloguing in Publication Data

Nutrition and disease.
  1. Nutrition
  I. Jarrett, R J
  612'.3   TX353

  ISBN 0-85664-561-3

Printed and bound in Great Britain by
Redwood Burn Ltd, Trowbridge and Esher

CONTENTS

PREFACE

Discussions and debates about food include its availability, cost and palatability — including the time-honoured recipe column in newspapers and journals — but increasingly they are concerned with the relation between food and health and disease. In this context the general public is addressed by a host of experts, many self-proclaimed and many who are banded together in committees. These, as well as the food freaks and faddists, advise on the beneficial or deleterious effects of this or that foodstuff, often presenting totally contradictory views which only serve to confuse the average man and woman who, not unnaturally, react by saying 'if the experts disagree I might as well eat what I like'. In affluent countries, of course, what they like may well be influenced by the widespread and pervasive advertising of the food industry. In less affluent countries people are only too happy to eat what they can get, though here too, cultural as well as economic factors influence dietary practices.

My purpose in editing this book is not to tell people what they should or should not eat but to provide a background of information about the relationships between nutrition and disease which should allow readers to put into context the statements, views and obiter dicta of others. This is not a textbook of nutrition nor of medicine, but an attempt to relate the two disciplines. I have attempted to avoid jargon, but have assumed some knowledge of biology in the reader. In fact the book is written with students of the various 'life sciences' in mind as the principal audience, though I hope that it will prove of interest to the educated layman as well.

The authors are not evangelists for any particular theory of nutrition but, like all human beings, have opinions. I have tried to ensure that opinions and facts are clearly recognisable one from another.

My own contribution to the book is concerned with the problems of 'overnutrition' and those associated with the refining of food. Dr Ebrahim, who has considerable experience in both Africa and South East Asia, deals with what is still the most widespread nutritional problem in the world — undernutrition — and Dr Poston brings us right up to date with a review of the relationship between food and immunological disorders, a branch of medicine which has developed enormously in the past decade. The toxicology of food is not considered as this will form part of the subject matter of our companion volume.

Preface

I would like to acknowledge the assistance of my daughter Penelope who not only drew the figures on pages 133 and 136 but also vetted my chapter for intelligibility.

INTRODUCTION

Much discussion of appropriate foods centres on what is 'natural',
and what sort of food man has adapted to during evolution. When one
considers the infinite variety of foods now used in the cuisine of
different countries and even the differences within a small country
such as Britain the task of compiling a list of 'natural' foods appears
superhuman. Perhaps more rewarding is an attempt to review the nature
of man's diet and its changes over the million years of his history, even
though much of this may be speculative.

The traditional anthropological classification of man's technological
development is into five basic forms: hunting and gathering; herding;
horticulture; agriculture; and industrial technology. The appropriateness
of this classification is debated, but it will serve as the basis of the
present discussion.

Hunting and gathering was the sole form of subsistence for homo
sapiens until 10,000 years ago and societies depending on these methods
were fairly common until the early part of this century. The aboriginal
inhabitants of Australia were hunter-gatherers, as were the Eskimos,
the North American Indians and, to a large extent, the South American
Indians, though many of these also cultivated manioc. In general, this
form of subsistence was only capable of nurturing relatively small
numbers of people and, except where wild life was plentiful, the return
in terms of effort expended was not very great. There are few
remaining hunter-gatherer societies left, largely because their technology
cannot compete even with fairly primitive industrial technology. Most
nowadays live largely on vegetables and fruit with little animal food.
One such group is the Kung Bushmen who live in an isolated area of
northern Botswana and they have been studied by anthropologists and
doctors. One of the latter, Professor Truswell, has made the following
points about these people with regard to their nutrition:

1. They are rarely obese and, at the end of the dry season, tend to
   become undernourished and energy deficient.
2. Except after illness or injury they do not experience malnutrition.
3. Hypertension was non-existent and blood pressure levels did not rise
   with age, which is the usual experience in almost all other
   communities. The presumed explanation for this is the complete

lack of salt in the diet of the Bushmen.

4. Their plasma cholesterol levels were very low, averaging 120 mg/dl (= 3.0 mmol/L).[1] In this context it is interesting that the principal sources of animal protein were the wild buck and small animals, such as hare. These animals have little fat in their muscle and have predominantly polyunsaturated fatty acids in what fat there is. Of their vegetable diet, which accounted for over half their food energy, the largest single item was the mongongo nut, which is rich in linoleic acid, one of the polyunsaturated fatty acids.

5. Dental carries did not occur — though teeth did get worn down with age. Apart from occasional wild honey, they did not eat sugar.

In this group, the men went out hunting, but the supply of meat was intermittent. The women collected the vegetable food, often walking long distances with heavy loads, sometimes including a baby. Older women remained in the camp and did various chores, including the fetching of water, which might involve a lot of walking, as the water supply was some distance from the camp. Numbers were small and apparently stationary. Expectation of life was reasonably good, with infections and accidents as the major cause of death in the younger population.

Although we cannot be sure, for there are no written records and the archaeological evidence is scanty, this seems likely to be a fairly typical description of a hunter-gatherer society over the millennia. Some may have had it easier, where wild life and vegetation were abundant; but for others life may well have been even harder. If we are to invoke evolution in discussing the nutrition of modern man, it is this sort of diet to which man has been most exposed and to which, presumably, he is or, at least, was adapted. Cereals, the predominant source of energy in the world today, providing 25 per cent of energy needs even in affluent countries, are only about 10,000 years old, not long in the evolutionary time scale.

Herding is a rather more complicated method of exploiting the environment. Examples of animals herded include reindeer, goats, cattle, camels, horses, pigs and llama. Some groups have lived almost entirely on herding; others combined it with farming. The animals would provide dietary protein either directly or via milk and milk products.

An economy based on herding allows a larger and more dense population than hunter-gathering, but it also depends on movement, because the animals need fresh pasture and a water supply, both of which may be dependent on the season. Thus herding peoples tend to be nomadic or 'transhumant', which differs from nomadism in that the cycle of movement is an annual one, following the seasons. Thus some Lapps move their reindeer to the coastal areas in the winter and to the better mountain pastures in the summer. The major insecurity of the herding economy is clearly the possibility — and reality — of disease in the animals.

Horticulture and agriculture are differentiated by the use of the plough. Horticulture implies gardening with hand tools only and as a means of subsistence it involves continual hard work for both sexes. Though it allows a larger population than hunter-gathering and herding, it does require, under primitive conditions, some movement in order to allow old gardens to recover their fertility. It is also subject to the vagaries of the weather and to infestation.

The invention of the plough was the major event in man's nutritional history and, perhaps, in his social one as well for the agricultural economy which followed allowed the growth of population and the institution of the town and city. The great civilisations of Mesopotamia, of Egypt, of Ancient Greece and of South America all were based upon the economy of a fairly primitive agriculture. This stage of technical development is still the norm in much of the world today, providing a subsistence economy for what have been called 'peasant agriculturists'.

Agriculture is a seasonal occupation and produces seasonal crops, so that food has to be stored. It allows the more prosperous to overeat (and under-exert) and so to become obese. From the grain is produced alcohol, with all that that implies. And it also introduces its own insecurity to the society relying on a single crop as its main source of energy. Failure of the crop, be it grain in Egypt in the Biblical story, or potatoes in Ireland in 1845, brings famine. Failure of the monsoon rains has been a recurrent cause of famine in India, a recent example being in Bihar in 1967, when national and international relief saved millions from starvation. Another, more complex, hazard is the spectre of deficiency diseases due to reliance on a single staple food, which may not contain sufficient vitamins or protein, particularly for growing children. This is probably a modern hazard associated with the large increase in population in the subsistence economies of the Third World. With more people, there is less space per family, so that it is difficult to grow the mixed vegetables necessary for a balanced diet.

The Industrial Economy

As countries become industrialised fewer and fewer people actually produce food and the domestic and community economies become totally separated. Industrial economies rely on trade, part of which includes the movement of food, so that the consumer's range of choice is greatly increased. It has been increased still further by the activities of the food industry, which has not only removed the seasonal nature of the supply of some staples, e.g. peas, but has actually created new choices, including the foods of convenience. For babies, however, industrialisation is associated with one restriction of choice, for breast feeding becomes the exception rather than the rule.

This range of choice, however, is dependent upon the means to pay and for millions of people attracted or forced by economic necessity to the towns the means are absent. The sad condition of much of the world's urban proletariat is described by Barbara Ward.[2] She points out that this new migrant population, which is crowding into the towns of Asia, Africa and Latin America, has the worst of both worlds — old rural traditions are lost and not replaced by urban education. Mothers have to go out to work often leaving babies inadequately cared for. Available food is often of poor quality and may be contaminated with pathogens or chemicals. Alcoholism, disease and violence complete the sorry picture.

All this can coincide with pockets of affluence, a situation which creates its own nutritional problems, though of a much less acute nature. So far, our affluent societies have been free of crop failure — though we all felt the effects of the rise in prices when the Russian wheat crop failed a few years ago and their authorities had to buy large amounts from North America. Some of us may worry about our foods being contaminated with insecticides and food additives. But for most people food is not a 'problem'; in affluent societies it is only so to those who observe the modern epidemics — coronary heart disease, diabetes mellitus, obesity, gall stones, and cancer — and suspect that nutrition has some part to play in their genesis.

Notes

1. This compares with average values of over 200 mg daily in industrialised communities.
2. Barbara Ward, *The Home of Man* (André Deutsch, 1976).

1 THE PROBLEMS OF UNDERNUTRITION

G.J. Ebrahim

Introduction

Man needs food to provide energy for the body's essential physiological functions like respiration, circulation, metabolism and so on, for maintaining body temperature, for the growth and repair of the body's tissues, and for obtaining essential nutrients for the several biochemical processes essential in body metabolism. The food that he eats is vegetable or animal in origin, and in both forms the energy which it provides is basically solar energy which has been 'trapped' by photo-synthesis and stored in various organs of the plant. Man, in common with other species of the animal kingdom, obtains this energy either by consuming these parts of the plant, e.g. cereal or tuber, or secondarily by consuming animals or their products who live on plants.

In common with all living organisms, man obtains food by interaction with his environment. Prior to the development of agriculture man was a hunter-gatherer and ate what his environment provided. Several tribes in Africa, the aborigines of Australia and the Eskimo are still by and large in this stage of development and their means of obtaining food from the environment can be described by the model in Figure 1.1 below. With the beginning of agriculture, man evolved agricultural technology, social systems and cultural practices to enable him to inter-act with his environment singly or in groups in order to obtain a regular supply of food. Commerce and marketing has also been part of this

Figure 1.1: Obtaining Nutrients from the Environment — the Hunter-Gatherer Stage

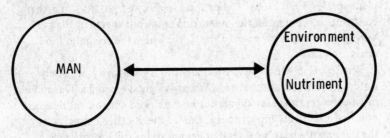

development and in recent years this aspect of food production has grown into 'agribusiness' which is concerned with the processing, sale and marketing of foods in different forms on national and even global scales. This aspect of man's interaction with his environment is demonstrated by the model in Figure 1.2.

Figure 1.2: Obtaining Nutrients from the Environment — the Complex Society

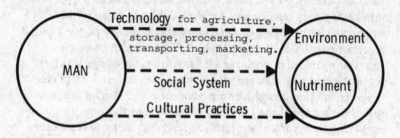

From the beginning of the practice of agriculture, there has been a tendency to concentrate on those species of plants that are most productive and rewarding in terms of labour (and capital) invested. In the past few centuries this trend has accelerated, especially with the coming of industrialisation and the development of cash economies. The supermarkets and convenience foods have further restricted choice in diets in urban industrial societies and through the development of multinational corporations are exerting their influence on Third World countries as well. This trend for more and more people to be nourished by fewer varieties of plants has reached the stage where a large proportion of the world's population is dependent on a handful of plant species. Four crops — wheat, rice, maize and potato — together constitute more than all the other food crops put together. Figures 1.3-1.5 show the main parts of the world where the common food crops are raised.

The forms in which we know many foods today may be totally different from their progenitors. Wheat is a good example. Three kinds of wheat were originally domesticated from wild grasses. All three are obsolete and hardly grown today. One of these, called emmer, was the dominant wheat for several millennia and is still grown on an appreciable scale in Ethiopia and parts of south India. Emmer was the

Figure 1.3: Principal Sources of Maize

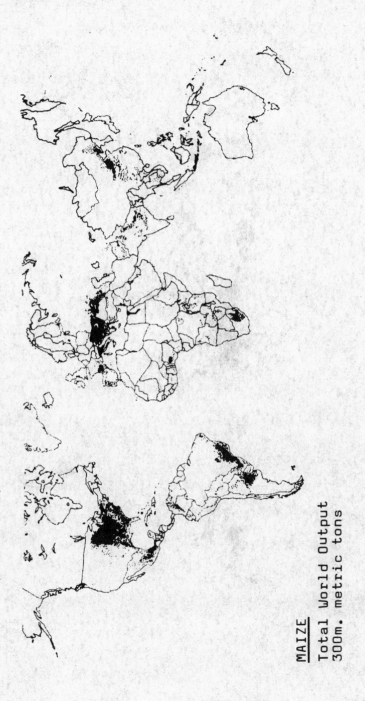

MAIZE
Total World Output
300m. metric tons

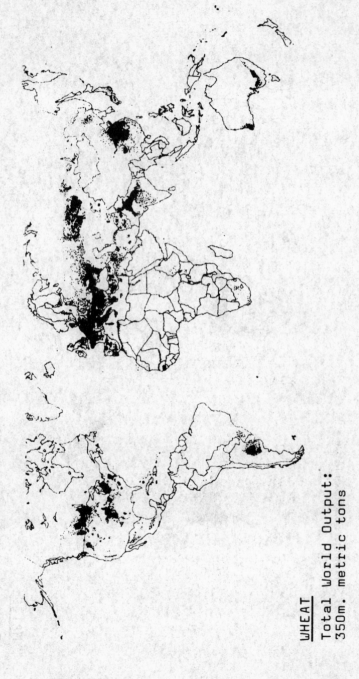

Figure 1.4: Principal Sources of Wheat

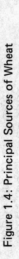

WHEAT
Total World Output:
350m. metric tons

Figure 1.5: Principal Sources of Rice

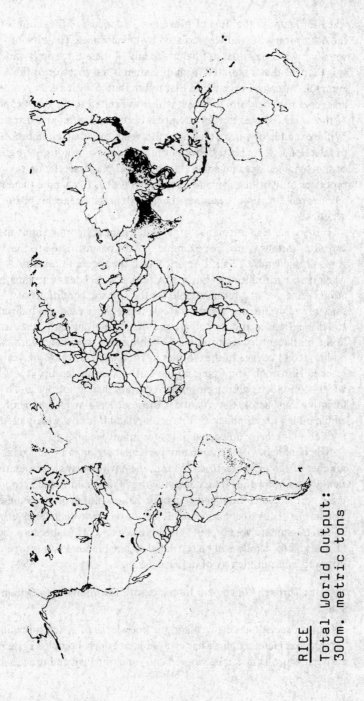

RICE
Total World Output:
300m. metric tons

wheat of Egypt at the time of Alexander's conquest of that country in the 4th century BC and was replaced by bread wheat. The type of wheat grown today does not belong to any of these three early varieties. It is thought that a mutated form of emmer is the ancestor of the common 'macaroni wheat' and that hybridisation with a wild goat grass gave rise to a form of wheat which was suited to the dry steppes of the world. Besides the selection that occurs in nature, as illustrated by the example of wheat, man also intervenes by a deliberate process of selection, e.g. by his taste for glutinous or non-glutinous, long-grained or short-grained rice and so on. It is now possible to accelerate the processes of hybridisation and selection as well as to channel them in any desired direction because of the growth in the science of plant genetics.

History has also intervened in several instances to bring about the spread of various crops. For example, potato was restricted to the Andean Highlands of South America until the sixteenth century when it was introduced to Europe. After a few decades of acclimatisation it emerged in a form suitable for the climatic conditions of Europe and eventually became a staple food. Sugar cane was indigenous to Asia and was introduced all around the Mediterranean by the Arabs in the ninth century. Christopher Columbus took specimens with him on his second voyage to the Antilles in 1493 and the following year it reached Hispaniola and Cuba. By the early sixteenth century it was widely consumed, with sugar refineries established in Europe and a lucrative trade across the Atlantic. Cottonseed as a major source of edible oil is a development of this century and it is now widely used as a 'filler' oil in many powdered milks for infant feeding.

The dominance of a crop in any particular region is a result of a number of ecological factors. The soil, the environmental temperature, rainfall and number of hours of sunlight will determine which crop will grow best. Socio-cultural and economic factors also depend on these. The farmer tends to concentrate his labour on a proven low-risk crop and to minimise diversity, but this also has its problems, because the farmer and his family will be restricted to one predominant source of nutrients and run the risk of deficiencies.

Systems Through Which Man Interacts with Environment to Obtain Food

As human society has evolved and the knowledge of agriculture and farming has increased, man has evolved increasingly complex systems through which land can be worked and food obtained and processed for use. At one end of the spectrum is the traditional farming system, characteristic of the peasant societies of the Third World. Such a system involves only man, his animals, his seed and his land, with very little involvement of industry, government or commercial and other agencies. In such a system productivity of the land is limited by the fertility of the soil and the climate, and the family income largely depends on the amount of land that can be worked with family labour. At the other end of the spectrum is the mechanised farm which forms part of the 'agribusiness', producing large crop surpluses. To compare outputs in the two systems, the average Indian or Pakistani farmer harvests little more than one metric ton of rice or wheat per hectare against 6 metric tons in the USA.

Agricultural Technology

Many of the farming systems of the developing world use a minimum of technology. Human muscle or draught animals provide the force for working the land. External inputs in the forms of machines, fuels and fertilisers are minimal or non-existent. The fertility of the soil is a limiting factor in output, particularly with regard to the nitrogen content, in which tropical soils tend to be deficient. The local varieties of grain grown are particularly suited to the environment, having been bred over a period of thousands of years, though the output is low. The traditional systems represent a type of ecological equilibrium which can be sustained indefinitely, given the available resources and provided that population growth is kept within the capacity of the system. On the other hand modernisation in agriculture needs heavy inputs in the form of energy, fertilisers, irrigation and high maintenance and research costs.

Much of agriculture in the Third World is rain-dependent. In a system where, because of low production, the margin of safety is low, a deficiency of even 25 per cent in rainfall can lead to crop failure of sufficient intensity to give rise to a threat of famine. In many parts of Asia and Africa such a deficiency in rainfall occurs on average once in five years.

Extension programmes specifically developed to help the small land holders and involving minimal capital expenditure are necessary to improve agricultural outputs in the developing world. The 'gardening' system of agriculture, like intercropping (more than one crop in the field), multiple cropping (several crops in succession in a year), relay planting (sowing a second crop between the rows of an earlier maturing crop), together with composting and irrigation through wells, need to be developed in order to improve food production in regions which suffer from chronic hunger.

Social Systems

Besides agricultural technology, social systems determine the amount of food available to an individual and his family. Inadequate nutrition has often been desribed as a *social* disease and in countries where malnutrition is common, its causes include factors inherent in the very nature of the society. Similarly, in countries where malnutrition has been overcome rapidly, political improvements have been major contributory factors.

In the typical developing country 50 to 80 per cent of the population is rural. The source of livelihood is the production of food or fibre crops or animal husbandry. The productivity of land is abysmally low; furthermore the ratio of land to population is dwindling. Thus in India the average size of a holding is 7.5 acres, but about 70 per cent of all holdings are below this average. Twenty-two per cent of rural families own no land at all and 47 per cent own less than an acre. The land tenure system in many countries favours the big landlord who employs farm labour at low wages. In one study of rural poverty in India it was found that 40 per cent of the rural population had an annual per capita consumer expenditure below the estimated breadline.

The rural poor have limited access to health care and education. Housing is substandard and life expectancy is low. Many are tied to a life of drudgery, eking out an existence on meagre land resources. In many such traditional agricultural systems almost half the energy derived by people and animals from the photosynthetic product of plants is expended to grow and prepare food, leaving little margin for anything else.

At the international level, the social system also tends to favour the rich. Many countries in Africa and Asia are former colonies in which the best land was principally utilised for the production of cash crops. Fifty-five per cent of crop land in the Philippines and over 80 per cent in Mauritius is assigned to cash crops. Moreover the thrust of agricultural research was also towards cash crops and local food crops were neglected. There are numerous centres for research on coffee, cocoa, oil palm, jute, rubber and cotton, but few for wheat, rice, maize and legumes. In more recent times the inequality of the international social system has taken yet another turn. The rising affluence of the industrialised nations has brought about a change in eating habits, causing an increased demand for meat and dairy products. This in turn has led to an increased demand for grain as cattle feed. In North America the per capita consumption of grain is about 1000 kg per year; of this, only about 75 kg are used directly as human food, much of the remainder being fed to animals. By contrast, cereal consumption in the Third World is about 200 kg per year, most of it being used as human food.

Cultural Factors

Agriculture has evolved with man and his culture. Since growing food is the main productive activity of rural areas, the agricultural systems used are very much part of the culture of a people. Thus there are several cultures in which cattle and especially the bull are given great importance. Land and its productivity are important in many peasant societies of tropical Africa. The festivities and carnivals in all rural societies are related to farming activities, e.g. spring festivals (to invoke fertility) and summer harvest festivals (for thanksgiving and rejoicing).

Cultural practices also determine how the land will be worked. For example, in some parts of Africa which grow cash crops, men work the plot of land set aside for the cash crop and women work on a separate family plot to grow food. The *type* of work may also be divided according to sex. Men hoe (or plough) the land and sow while women do the weeding and harvesting.

Religion and culture often determine the choice of foods. Many communities classify foods as 'hot' and 'cold' and avoid food combinations that are thought to be deleterious. The caste system in India determines not only the types of food that an individual may eat or abstain from, but also the person who may cook the food, the person(s) with whom he may take food and the rituals to be followed at meals.

In addition to the 'hot' and 'cold' classification there are 'light' foods to be eaten during illnesses, there are celebration foods for specific festivals (e.g. the Christmas turkey in the West, the Onam festival of Kerala, India which is celebrated with 22 varieties of preparations from root vegetables), there are foods which people abstain from on certain days (e.g. meat on Fridays) and there are foods for entertaining important visitors.

From the nutritional point of view, cultural practices are more important in the case of certain vulnerable groups. In most societies food taboos and practices are directed at the pregnant woman and her child. In many cultures the pregnant woman is advised to eat less so

that she will have an easy labour. Lamb meat and eggs are not allowed
throughout pregnancy because of their supposed effects on the fetus.
Similarly, there are several weaning practices which are harmful to the
infant, e.g. abrupt weaning by separating the infant from the mother,
the type of food introduced, the form and composition of the weaning
foods offered, etc.

The various beliefs and dietary practices of a community are one of
the many predisposing factors in malnutrition. An important
precipitating factor in most instances is infection. The nutritional needs
of the body are increased during an episode of illness, when the
appetite is often decreased: in addition, various foods are withheld in
the mistaken belief that such a practice hastens recovery. The practice
of 'starving a cold' is well known. Similarly, food is often withheld from
a child suffering from diarrhoea, measles and other febrile illnesses. The
effect of bad dietary practices is greatest during bouts of illness, when
the nutritional status of the individual deteriorates rapidly.

Storage and Utilisation of Food

The crop which is harvested is stored and processed before it is cooked
and eaten. During each of these steps nutrients may be altered. For
example, if storage facilities are inadequate, much of the foodgrain may
be lost to insects and rodents. In some cases the losses may amount to
almost a third of the total crop. Food can also deteriorate during storage
because of fungal growth caused by temperature and humidity and lack
of aeration. Thus aflatoxin can affect both ground nuts and other food
crops, resulting in health hazards to the consumers.

Apart from vegetables and fruits, most food crops are processed
before eating. The aim of such processing is to reduce bulk, improve
digestibility, improve appearance, add flavours and increase palatability.
Many methods of processing also help the keeping qualities of the crop,
so that it can be stored for a prolonged period of time.

The commonest form of processing is milling, either for altering
flavour or for polishing, as in the case of rice. In the case of both, the
outer layers of the grain are discarded as bran. All nutrients are not
evenly distributed in the grain. For example, the two outer layers
[Aleurone and Scutellum (Figure 1.6)] comprise 8.5 per cent of the
weight of the grain and contain 94 per cent of Thiamine, 51 per cent of
Riboflavin, 83 per cent of Niacin and 21 per cent of the protein
of the grain. The highly refined flour or polished rice can be made into
attractive white bread or cooked white rice, but will be devoid of
nutrients as well as fibre and consist principally of starch. In most rural

Figure 1.6: Diagram of Longitudinal Section of Cereal Grain

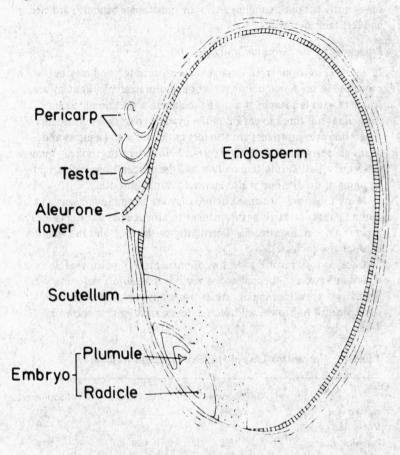

societies home pounding or stone grinding, with or without prior fermenting, is the common method of preparing flour from the cereal, but the method is time-consuming and laborious and the flour is coarse and gritty, so that it is gradually being abandoned in favour of the village mill.

Parboiling of rice is a processing method used in some of the rural areas where rice is a staple food. It has been estimated that more than a sixth of the rice consumed is treated by parboiling. The grain is soaked, steamed and dried carefully. During the soaking, nutrients pass from the outer into the inner parts of the grain and the germ becomes more firmly attached during drying. Because of this, the grain loses fewer nutrients during milling. Also the outer coats become hardened and resistant to insects.

Processing in the Home and the Kitchen

In addition to commercial or large-scale processing, food may be processed in the home before it is cooked. For example, in many areas where cassava is a staple, it must be soaked in water, pounded and washed several times to get rid of the cyanide toxins present in the tuber; however, nutrients are also lost in the process. Legumes and beans are germinated until they sprout before they are cooked. Vitamin C is synthesised during germination and the concentration of certain vitamins of the B group is also increased during sprouting.

Many foods are fermented before they are eaten. Soya beans and ground nuts are treated in this manner to produce pastes or cheese. The process helps to improve the digestibility of the food and the vitamin content also increases.

Cooking may involve some loss of nutrients, e.g. when vegetables are boiled in water and then all excess water is drained off before serving. Similarly, excess washing of cereals, especially rice to make it look white instead of brown, will result in loss of nutrients as shown in Table 1.1.

Table 1.1: Percentage Loss of Nutrients through Washing

	Thiamine	Riboflavin	Nicotinic acid
Husked rice	21%	8%	13%
Milled rice	20%	26%	23%
Parboiled rice	15%	15%	13%
Home pounded rice	7%	12%	10%

During cooking various foods absorb water at different rates, producing different amounts of bulk. The caloric density, i.e. the number of calories per unit volume of food eaten, is important especially in children and other vulnerable groups in communities subsisting on marginal nutrition. Thus both rice and potato absorb water in differing proportions so that the calories or protein per 100 grams of cooked rice or creamed potato are very different from those in the raw foods.

Table 1.2: Effects of Boiling Potato and Rice

	Percentage of water		Protein/100 g of cooked product	
	Raw	Boiled	Raw	Boiled
Potato	76%	81%	2.1	1.4
Rice	12%	70.88%	6.8	2.3—1.0

The Food Industry

Rapid urbanisation and affluence have created a demand for pre-cooked and convenience foods, with supermarket chains and a variety of industry and business interests providing the supply of such foods. This 'agribusiness' has spawned giant multinationals with business interests extending from farm machinery and fertilisers to packaging and shipping of the finished products. In many cases there is over-enthusiastic promotion of the packaged foods which influences eating habits even in well-informed societies. Between 1959 and 1970, the consumption of fruit and vegetables declined in the US by more than a fifth. Consumption of milk dropped 20 per cent, while that of soft drinks went up 79 per cent. The sales of potato crisps went up 85 per cent, and ice cream 29 per cent. Processed convenience food does not necessarily give the customer the best value for money. For example, corn costing US $2.95 a bushel when processed into Cocoa Puffs (corn meal, sugar, corn syrup, cocoa, salt, etc) fetches $75 a bushel, and puffed wheat under the name of Quaker Oats fetches $110 per bushel. There is also the added hint that such products have captured the 'goodness of sunshine' and are health promoting! The effects of such promotion are seen at their maximum in rural areas of the developing countries where white bread, coca-cola and biscuits have become prestige items, and scant family resources are being spent on food items with little nutritive value.

This brief outline of the social, cultural, technical and commercial factors in the production and utilisation of food provides a background against which nutritional deficiencies occur in individuals, families and communities. In their turn nutritional deficiencies affect the health of the people concerned. The following pages describe the prevalence of individual nutritional disorders, their relationship to health, and discuss methods of prevention.

Nutrition in Pregnancy and the Growth of the Fetus

In all mammals, anatomical and physiological changes occur in the body of the mother during pregnancy to create a suitable environment for the growth of the fetus. A complex series of endocrinological and metabolic changes also take place which facilitate the handling of nutrients by the body tissues of the mother as well as their transfer to the fetus.

The fetus is comparatively small in the early stages of pregnancy, even though there is rapid cellular multiplication and differentiation. It is not until the third trimester[1] that fetal growth is such that nutrients are required in appreciable quantities. Studies in healthy and under-nourished women show that, up to the last trimester, there is very little difference in fetal weight between the two groups. Significant changes in birthweight occur mainly between the twenty-fifth and fortieth weeks of pregnancy.

Effects of the Previous Health and Nutritional Status of the Mother

The growth of the fetus can be regarded as a result of the interaction between its genetic potential and the intrauterine environment. Mothers who enter pregnancy in good health, with sound reproductive physiology, and who have not suffered ill health or nutritional deprivation in childhood will have larger and healthier infants than mothers who do not have such advantages. Thus, there is a significant difference in average birthweights between babies born in affluent societies and those born in the developing countries. Within a society birth weights tend to be higher in the upper socio-economic groups compared with the lower, and this is in keeping with the differences in several other health indices in the groups.

Weight at birth is also influenced by factors operating during pregnancy. Serious illnesses, complications of pregnancy, nutritional deprivation, emotional and psychological stress can all influence the growth of the fetus through their adverse effect on the mother, or by interfering with placental growth and transport of nutrients to the fetus.

Fetal Growth

Our knowledge of the nutritional requirements of growth in the human fetus has developed from a variety of studies. The relationship between food intake in the mother and its effect on the offspring is best seen in animal experiments, especially in those species where the period of gestation is relatively short and a correlation between dietary intake and fetal growth can be readily seen. There have been epidemiological studies in women comparing birth weights in different social groups and similar observations during famine and war, which show the effects of acute food shortages on fetal growth. All such studies indicate that most of the growth in the size of the fetus occurs in the latter part of pregnancy. For example, at the end of the third month of gestation, the fetus weighs approximately 30 g. By comparison, towards the end of gestation the fetus is daily laying down 500 mg of nitrogen (equivalent to 3 g of body tissue), over 300 mg calcium and 200 mg phosphorus. The maximum rate of fetal growth is during 32-38 weeks of pregnancy, when the weight virtually doubles.

Nutritional Requirements of the Fetus

Proteins

The placenta transports protein primarily as amino acids which are then synthesised by the fetus into tissue proteins. Nitrogen balance studies during pregnancy in healthy English women show an average excess of intake over loss of 92 g; since 50 g are needed for the growth of fetal and placental tissues, there is a margin of safety of 42 g, or 45 per cent. By comparison, dietary studies in undernourished Indian women indicate that they have a safety margin of only 6 g, or 12 per cent.

Fat

Most of the 350 g of fetal body fat is deposited between the thirty-fifth and fortieth weeks of pregnancy, about half of this between the thirty-fifth and thirty-eighth weeks. In the early stages of gestation there is no fat laid down apart from essential lipids and phospholipids for the central nervous system and the cell-walls. Until the middle of gestation, there is only about 0.5 per cent fat in the body of the fetus, after which the amount increases, reaching 7.8 per cent at thirty-four weeks of gestation and 16 per cent before birth. During the last month of intrauterine life as much as 14 g of fat per day is laid down. Of this, placental transport of fatty acids accounts for 40 per cent of fetal fat; the remainder is synthesised by the fetus.

Carbohydrate

The fetus has about 9 g of carbohydrate at thirty-three weeks of gestation, and at birth it rises to 34 g. The concentration of glycogen in the liver and skeletal muscles increases during the latter part of gestation as shown in Table 1.3.

Table 1.3: Concentration of Carbohydrate (g per 100 g)

Maturity (weeks)	Heart	Liver	Muscle
31	0.76	0.98	1.63
40	1.01	3.92	2.67

The Role of the Placenta

The placenta plays an important role in the transfer of nutrients from
the mother to the fetus. It is not just an organ of simple transport, but
is able to take up nutrients selectively and either process or re-synthesise
them before they reach the fetus. The supply of nutrients to the
growing fetus depends upon both the amount of maternal blood flowing
through the placenta as well as the food substances carried by it. The
efficiency with which the placenta can concentrate, synthesise and
transport essential nutrients will also determine the food supply to the
fetus.

Factors which regulate fetal growth also regulate the growth of the
placenta. Thus the metabolic work of the placenta depends upon the
growth capabilities of the fetus and not the other way around. Fetal
malnutrition commonly arises from either an insufficient supply from
the mother due to some vascular abnormality of the placenta, or from
nutritional deficiency in the mother, and only occasionally from
reduced placental transport of nutrients. The nature, timing and duration
of nutritional deficit is thought to account for the different degrees of
intrauterine growth retardation expressed as different forms of fetal
malnutrition. It has been estimated that in a third to a half of 'small
for dates' infants (i.e. with birth weight less than 2500 g) the period of
gestation is actually more than thirty-seven weeks; thus, the reduction
in birth weight is due to growth retardation rather than immaturity.

Mechanism of Placental Transfer

Various parts of the placenta are actively involved in the transfer,
processing and synthesis of nutrients under the influence of maternal,
fetal and placental hormones. Gases and water diffuse freely across
the placenta, but the mechanism of transport for other substances is
not understood. The gradient is not directly from maternal to fetal
blood, but from maternal blood to the maternal side of the placenta,

where proteins, enzymes, nucleic acids, etc. may be synthesised. Further conversion and synthesis occurs in the fetal part of the placenta. Carbohydrate is the principal metabolic fuel of the fetus and is provided in continuous supply by transfer of glucose from the mother through the placenta. On the other hand, fat is not a main source of energy in the fetus, so there is only a slow limited transfer of fatty acids across the placenta. Cell growth in the fetus is assumed to result from fetal synthesis of proteins from the amino acids transferred through the placenta.

Nutrition of the Mother

The state of the mother's physiology, especially reproductive physiology, at the time when she commences a pregnancy has considerable influence on the growth of the fetus. Several studies provide evidence for the relationship between adult size, reproductive efficiency and socio-economic status. In general, the baby of a short woman is lighter and has less vitality and a lower survival than that of a tall woman. Stunting in the mother cannot be overcome by a good diet in pregnancy and the same applies to reproductive efficiency. It is axiomatic that preparation for pregnancy should begin with good nutrition and health care in *childhood* so that women enter motherhood having achieved optimal growth and health. For many years it has been known that the height of the mother is closely related to birth weight and pregnancy outcome and this was amply demonstrated in surveys of perinatal mortality in the UK in 1958 and 1970. These surveys have also revealed that there are more short mothers in the lower socio-economic groups, which means that inadequate nutrition and larger number of illnesses prevent many girls in this social group from achieving optimal physique. They are thus at a disadvantage as regards childbearing. Similar studies in the United States, conducted by the National Institute of Health, have shown that mothers who weigh more than 150 lbs (68 kg) at conception or who gain more than 30 lbs (13.6 kg) in weight during pregnancy tend to have larger and healthier babies with a lower perinatal mortality than those of mothers who weigh less or gain less weight than above.

Weight Gain in Pregnancy

Dietary studies in well-nourished women in Aberdeen showed that the average weight gain during pregnancy was 12.5 kg, including 3.5 kg laid down as fat in the mother, representing an energy store of 30,000 kcal (Table 1.4). The gain in weight follows a general pattern:

(i) Minimal accumulation (almost all in 'maternal compartment')
in the first trimester   1 kg
(ii) Approximately 0.3 kg per week (of which 60 per cent is in the
'maternal compartment') in the second trimester   3 kg
(iii) About 0.3 to 0.5 kg per week (of which 60 per cent is in the
'fetal compartment') in the third trimester   6 kg

The gain in weight related to the products of conception occurs mostly
in the latter part of pregnancy, whereas that attributable to maternal
storage is dispersed more evenly throughout the course of pregnancy.

More recently calorimetric and metabolic studies have confirmed the
above observations. The mean daily increase in energy intake in a
healthy and well-nourished woman is just over 100 calories for the
whole period of pregnancy, with a median value of 9 calories for the
first trimester, 84 for the second and 216 for the third. In most cases
the addition of 12 ounces of milk to a well-balanced diet which
maintains a normal pregnant woman in constant weight is sufficient to
meet all the extra energy requirements of pregnancy.

Table 1.4: Compartments of Weight Gain in Pregnancy

	Cumulative gain (kg) at end of each trimester		
	1	2	3
Fetal compartment			
Fetus	Negligible	1.0	3.4
Placenta	Negligible	0.3	0.6
Amniotic fluid	Negligible	0.4	1.0
Total		1.7	5.0
Maternal compartment			
Increased size of uterus	0.3	0.8	1.0
Increased breast size	0.1	0.3	0.5
Increased blood volume	0.3	1.3	1.5
Increased extracellular fluid	0	0	1.5
Total	0.7	2.4	4.5
Total gain accounted for	0.7	4.1	9.5
Usual gain in weight			12.5 kg
Difference as body fat			3.0 kg

Iron and Folic Acid Requirements

Pregnancy imposes a considerable strain on the maternal blood forming system. In most instances the greatest need is for iron and to a lesser extent for folic acid. The amount of elemental iron in a fetus at birth is approximately 300 mg and the quantity required for increased red cell formation in the mother to prevent anaemia in the face of increased plasma volume is 500 mg. In other words, the requirement for iron during pregnancy is slightly less than 1 g, concentrated for the most part in the last half of gestation.

In an adequate diet the daily iron content is 10-15 mg, of which 10 to 20 per cent is absorbed. Dietary iron will thus provide just a little more than the requirement so that other sources of iron are needed. Body stores of iron, mainly in the bone marrow, are available, but frequently the amount is not sufficient to meet the demand. Iron stores in healthy young American women average 300 mg. However, a significant number of women enter pregnancy with depleted or no iron stores because of previous pregnancies or menstrual loss. The relatively small amounts of iron in the diet and the low stores of iron are not enough to meet the greatly increased requirements of iron for the synthesis of maternal and fetal haemoglobin. Thus, anaemia is a relatively common complication of pregnancy, even in developed countries.

Anaemia of pregnancy is common in all developing countries. In a collaborative study involving seven Latin American countries, iron deficiency was present in 48 per cent of pregnant women as compared with 21 per cent of non-pregnant women. Similar prevalence studies have shown that 15-50 per cent of women in Africa, and more than 20 per cent of women in Asia have haemoglobin levels below 10 g/dl mostly due to iron deficiency.

Maternal anaemia is associated with an increased risk of low birth weight and perinatal death. In one study in East Africa it was found that among mothers whose haemoglobin was 7.4 g/dl or less at the time of delivery the incidence of low birth weight ($<$ 2,500 g) was 42 per cent and the stillbirth rate was 147.1 per 1,000. In mothers with haemoglobin of 8.8 g/dl and above the incidence of low birth weight was 12.7 per cent and stillbirths 51.0 per 1,000. Similarly, in Malaysia it has been reported that in mothers with a haemoglobin of 6.5 g/dl or less the incidence of low birth weight was 20 per cent compared to 7 per cent in non-anaemic pregnancies and the perinatal loss in the anaemic mothers was more than twice that of the non-anaemic ones.

Recommended Allowances

Studies on the energy costs of pregnancy indicate that about 100 calories per day extra are required for the entire gestation period. These are not evenly distributed but more or less follow the pattern of fetal growth and maternal weight gain. For example, energy balance is maintained by the addition of 10 calories per day in the first trimester, ₋5 in the second and 220 in the third.

The protein requirement is related to energy intake. Most balance studies show a linear relation between calorie intake and nitrogen balance. The average nitrogen retention during pregnancy is 51 ± 40 mg/kg per day at the average intake of 52 ± 9 calories and 1.7 g protein per kg body weight daily.

Based on the above considerations the World Health Organisation has recommended an intake of 1.01 g/kg protein and 46 kcalories/kg for the average woman with a body weight of 55 kg. These recommendations are general and tend to err on the safe side. Most countries have made specific recommendations in relation to their individual circumstances and national dietary patterns (Table 1.5).

Table 1.5: Daily Protein and Energy Allowances for Women in Several Countries

Country (year)	Reference body weight (kg)	Protein (g/kg) Non-pregnant	Protein (g/kg) Pregnant	Energy kcal/kg Non-pregnant	Energy kcal/kg Pregnant
Canada (1974)	56	0.70	0.85	43	52
Colombia (1955)	55	1.09	1.31	36	40
Guatemala (1969)	55	1.18	2.36	36	40
India (1968)	45	1.00	1.22	49	56
Philippines (1970)	49	1.12	1.32	39	47
United Kingdom (1969)	55	1.00	1.09	40	44
United States (1968)	53	0.95	1.12	34	42

Source: Modified from Calloway, D.H. in M. Winnick (ed.), *Nutrition and Foetal Development* (J. Wiley and Sons, New York, 1976).

As regards iron and folic acid, it has been found that diets which provide the recommended amounts of protein and calories from a mixture of foods will also provide sufficient iron and folic acid. However, to *ensure* adequate intake it is necessary to take additional iron and folic acid especially in the last trimester.

Effects of Nutritional Deficiency in Pregnancy

Several investigations in laboratory animals show that restricting food in pregnancy can have profound effects on the physiological adjustments in the mother, as well as on the growth and development of the fetus. The effects of restricting only calories cannot be separated from those of restricting proteins, because the body can burn proteins to provide energy; conversely, calories have a protein-sparing effect. Generally speaking in most laboratory animals food deficiency in pregnancy reduces the size of the litter, the weight of the individual young and the survival rate. Subsequent growth of the offspring is also affected, though it is more so when food deficiency extends into the period of lactation.

More recent studies of the cellular mechanisms of growth have measured the DNA content of an organ as an index of cell number and the protein content as an index of cell size. These studies demonstrate that the growth of an organ takes place in phases. There is at first an increase in the number of cells followed by an increase in the size of the individual cell. Food restriction at the time of cell division can significantly affect the size of an organ, and conceivably such a restriction of growth is irreversible.

In the human there are problems in the interpretation of the effects of dietary deficiency on the fetus. In the poorer parts of the world, food deficiency during pregnancy is the rule, but comparisons with the more affluent societies are difficult because of the genetic, socio-economic and other differences. In the case of Western Europe, however, some information is available from 'experiments of nature' like famine and war. During the last war, acute food shortage reaching famine proportions occurred on two separate occasions. The siege of Leningrad lasted 18 months (from August 1941 to January 1943) and for a period of six months (September 1941 to February 1942) conditions were extremely severe. Two periods of food deficiency can be identified, a time when there was a generally increasing restriction of food and later, a period of *extreme* deficiency when the diet consisted mainly of bread, one half of it made up of defective rye flour and the rest consisting of cellulose, malt and bran. During the early part of the siege, the average birth weight decreased significantly. It was found that 49 per cent of those born in the first half of 1942 (thus having suffered nutritional deprivation in the last trimester of pregnancy) weighed less than 2,500 g. There were, of course, other potential contributing factors like excessive physical exertion, lack of rest, nervous tension, extremes of cold, etc.

A similar period of famine was also experienced in Holland in the winter of 1944 to 1945. The period of food shortage was more sharply demarcated than in the case of Leningrad and overwork and other strains were not so prominent. The famine reached its maximum severity after six weeks and lasted for 27 weeks altogether. Thus, pregnant women were exposed to nutritional deprivation for varying lengths of time, but none was exposed for the whole gestation period. Birth weights were lowest in the case of those mothers who had experienced 18 to 21 weeks of famine and began to rise immediately after the famine ended. Lowest median birth weights were reached when exposure to famine was in the second half of pregnancy. Exposure very early in pregnancy did not affect the birth weight. Infants born of mothers who had conceived in the latter part of the famine, so that their babies experienced 27 weeks of gestation during the famine and an average of 9 weeks after it ended, attained a higher mean birth weight than those born in the early part of the famine.

In the developing world, food shortage is chronic and is often acute during times of poor harvests. In a dietary survey of 352 pregnant women in India it was found that the mean daily intake was 1,402 kcalories and 38 g protein. Many women in the lower socio-economic groups enter pregnancy after a childhood in which undernutrition and recurrent illnesses are common, so that they have not obtained the optimum in growth and physiological development. Thus, the mean body weight in 498 non-pregnant Indian women in the low socio-economic group was found to be only 42.4 kg. Moreover, on their marginal nutrition many pregnant women gain very little weight. In one study of 48 pregnant women, the mean gain in body weight from the twelfth to the fortieth week of pregnancy was 6.02 kg. In another study of 130 pregnant women, almost half failed to gain weight between the thirty-second and thirty-sixth weeks and thereafter. Besides poor weight gain many show clinical signs of nutritional deficiency. In a nutritional survey carried out amongst 198 pregnant women during the third trimester of pregnancy, 44 per cent showed clinical signs of Vitamin B complex deficiency, 9.5 per cent had oedema of the legs and 14.5 per cent showed signs of lack of Vitamin A. The mean birth weight in such women from the lower socio-economic group was 2,778 g as compared to 3,055 g in the higher social group.

A survey of dietary intake of women in coastal Tanzania revealed that mean daily energy intake was 1,850 kcalories and that of protein was 51.5 g. Iron intake in the diet ranged from 10 to 16.2 mg per day. A significant correlation was seen between the energy intake of the mother and the size of the baby. In order to have a baby weighing more than 3.1 kg it was necessary that the mother should consume at least 50 g of protein daily. Forty per cent of the women were eating less protein than this amount. Energy deficiency was a much more serious problem. To have a baby weighing 3.1 kg a mother had to consume 2,200 calories per day, and only 20 per cent of the women had as much.

A similar study in four Guatemalan villages showed that the mean intake of calories and protein during pregnancy was 1,500 calories and 40 g respectively. The average maternal height in rural Guatemala is 149 cm which is 12 cm less than the average height for women in a sample of the white population in the USA. Much of this low maternal height is accounted for by growth retardation during the first seven years of life. The average weight gain in pregnancy was 7 kg, which is about half of that in well-nourished women in affluent societies. Predictably, the mean birth weight was low at 3 kg and of 39 infants with normal gestational age about a third weighed 2.5 kg or less. Dietary histories again indicated a close assocation between food intake and the weight of the baby at birth. For example, in 34 women with a daily caloric intake of 700 to 1,800, the mean birth weight was 2.8 kg. In eight women with a daily caloric intake of 1,900 to 2,100 calories the mean birth weight was 3 kg and in 9 women with a daily caloric intake to 2,200 to 3,100 calories the mean birth weight was 3.2 kg. Supplementation studies showed that the total caloric intake was a more critical variable than protein, and the incidence of lighter babies was highest when the Guatemalan mother consumed less than 1,800 calories per day.

Cellular Growth in the Fetus

The organ and body weights of infants who were either still-born, or died in the neonatal period, were compared in 1002 consecutive necropsies in New York City. In the case of mothers from the low socio-economic groups, the body size of the infants as well as the weights of the brain, heart, liver, spleen, thymus, kidneys and adrenals were all significantly less than in the case of infants born to better-off mothers. The body weight was less by 13 to 17 per cent of the mean of infants born to well-to-do mothers. Amongst the organs the thymus, spleen and liver were found to be particularly small.

Measurements of DNA and DNA protein ratio in kidney, heart and liver of the human fetus indicate that these organs grow in several phases during intrauterine life:

(i) Between the fourteenth and twenty-fifth week of intrauterine life, the cells in all the three organs are dividing rapidly. The DNA content approximately doubles each week.

(ii) Between the thirtieth and fortieth weeks there is a rapid growth in cell size. The cells still increase in number, but more slowly.

(iii) At term all three organs still had less than 20 per cent of the numbers of cells characteristic of the adult.

In the case of babies who were 'small for dates' the protein/DNA ratio was normal, but the *total* DNA tended to be low.

Weight at Birth and Body Composition of the Fetus

When the body composition of still-born infants in undernourished Indian women was compared with that of similar infants of well-nourished English women, it was found that at 26-28 weeks of gestation the total body weights were similar in both groups, but there were significant qualitative differences. There was a deficit in protein and iron content in the case of Indian babies (Table 1.6).

Table 1.6: Fetal Body Composition in Undernourished Indian and Healthy English Women at Different Weights and Gestational Age

	Age (weeks)	Water (g)	Protein (g)	Fat (g)	Cu (g)	PO_4 (g)	Mg (mg)	Iron (mg)
Weight 1,000 g								
Indian[a]	27	862	80	26	5.8	3.3	200	59
English[b]	26	860	87.5	10	60	3.4	220	64
Weight 1,500 g								
Indian	34	1248	126	75	10.5	5.0	325	81
English	31	1270	156	35	10.0	5.6	350	100
Weight 2,000 g								
Indian	38	1604	176	148	14.6	8.6	425	108
English	33	1620	231	100	15.0	8.2	460	160
Weight 2,500 g								
Indian	40	1935	242	242	19.0	10.8	540	138
English	35	1940	306	185	20	11	580	220
Weight 3,000 g								
Indian	40	2238	291	366	22.7	11.4	655	165
English	38	2180	344	360	25.0	14.0	700	260

[a] Apte, S., and Iyengar, L. (1972), *Br. J. Nutn.,* vol. 27, p. 305.

[b] Widdowson, E.M. in N.S. Assali (ed.), *Biology of Gestation*, vol. 2, Academic Press, NY.

In the case of Indian fetuses, liver stores of Vitamin A, B_2 and folate were lower than those of infants of well-nourished mothers.

Effects of Supplementing Maternal Diet

In well-nourished communities no supplementation is necessary beyond the administration of iron and folic acid in the last trimester and the normal satisfaction of hunger from a mixed diet. In communities where diets are inadequate and where a large proportion of mothers enter reproduction after a childhood characterised by inadequate growth, supplementation is important to avoid fetal malnutrition. Repeated pregnancies in such a situation lead to depletion of maternal tissues and impaired reproductive efficiency. Several countries have now evolved national programmes for protecting the diets of pregnant and lactating women through a supply of free subsidised foods, especially milk, through fortification of ordinary foods to improve their nutritive value, and sometimes through cash benefits to improve purchasing power.

In developing countries, where health resources are meagre and a large number of families exist on marginal nutrition, it is necessary to identify the minimum supplementation necessary for adequate fetal growth. Studies in Guatemala have shown that supplementing the pregnant woman's diet by 233 kcalories per day led to a significant increase in fetal birth weight. Heavier babies were born to mothers who ingested more calories during pregnancy, irrespective of whether the calories were derived from the usual diet or from food supplements. The conversion of food calories into fetal tissues was at the rate of 3 g of baby per 1,000 kcalories of food. It was significant that in the same mother there was an average difference of 2.2 g between successive siblings per change of 1,000 kcalories in the diet. Though there are a host of factors which can influence birth weight, these findings emphasise the importance of adequate food intake during pregnancy. What is more important is the shift of emphasis from protein to calories. In most instances, when the energy requirement is satisfied by adequate food intake, the requirement of protein is also taken care of, unless the diet is bizarre.

More recent work in India adds yet another facet to the whole question of supplementation in pregnancy. When diets of Indian women in low socio-economic groups were supplemented with 50 g protein and 500 calories, the mean gain in weight by the mothers during pregnancy was 2.84 kg, significantly greater than the 1.02 kg in the control group; the mean birth weight of the babies (3,000 g) was also significantly greater than those of the controls (2,700 g).

Interestingly, when the supplement consisted of 30-60 mg iron and 200-500 mg of folic acid, instead of food, the mean birth weight was 2,880 g compared to 2,500 g in the controls and the incidence of babies weighing less than 2,300 g was 10 per cent as compared to 23 per cent in the control group. The placentas in the supplemented group were heavier and their DNA content was higher. It has been suggested that folic acid has a growth promoting action besides being a haemopoietic factor. On the basis of these studies, the government of India has commenced a national programme of supplementation with iron and folic acid for pregnant women.

Breast Feeding

All babies thrive on their mothers' milk. The period of neonatal life and early infancy is characterised by rapid growth, so that the average baby at four months of life weighs twice as much as at birth, and three times as much when six months old. This increase in growth includes increased muscle mass, growth of organs, expansion of blood volume and linear increase in the long bones. The nutrients required to sustain such a rapid growth are all supplied by breast milk alone in the first three to four months of life, in all infants. The composition of human milk should therefore provide a clue to the physiological needs for energy and nutrients in infants.

Protein Requirements

Various studies have been conducted to ascertain the requirements of proteins during infancy. In one type of study, infants were fed mixtures of amino acids in various combinations and the levels of individual amino acids which supported adequate growth were taken as the optimal levels. In another study, infants were fed a variety of milk formulae in quantities which maintained adequate growth and the concentration of each individual amino acid in the milk was then calculated to give the required amount. Using the data from these studies an Expert Committee of the World Health Organisation made recommendations on the amino acid requirement in infants (Table 1.7).

In adults, eight amino acids are essential. They cannot be synthesised in the body and must be supplied in food. These are isoleucine, leucine, lysine, methionine, phenylalanine, threonine, tryptophan and valine. Infants require these eight plus histidine. Precise information on the requirements of amino acids at different periods of

Table 1.7: Estimated Requirements of Essential Amino Acids

Amino acid	Amino acid mixture which will maintain adequate growth mg/kg/day[a]	Amino acid content of various milk formulae which will maintain adequate growth mg/kg/day[b]	Suggested pattern mg/gm protein[c]
Histidine	34	28	14
Isoleucine	119	70	35
Leucine	229	161	80
Lysine	103	161	52
Methionine and Cystine	45 + Cystine	58	29
Phenylalanine and Tyrosine	90 + Tyrosine	125	63
Threonine	87	116	44
Tryptophan	22	17	8.5
Valine	105	93	47

[a] Holt, L.E. and Syderman, S.E. in W.L. Nyan (ed.), *Amino acid metabolism and genetic variation* (McGraw-Hill, New York, 1967) p. 381.
[b] Fomon, S.J. and Filer, L.J.
[c] Joint FAO/WHO Expert Committee, 1973.

Table 1.8: Estimated Daily Intake of Energy, Protein and Essential Amino Acids at Different Ages

	1 month	2 months	3 months	6 months
Mean intake of breast milk	600 ml	727 ml	765 ml	780 ml
Calories	420	509	535	546
Protein (g)	6.4	7.7	8.2	8.3
Amino acids (mg)				
Histidine	186	225	237	241
Isoleucine	402	487	512	522
Leucine	720	872	918	936
Lysine	540	654	688	702
Methionine	114	138	145	148
Phenylalanine	288	348	367	374
Threonine	348	421	443	452
Tryptophan	180	218	229	234
Valine	522	632	665	678

growth in the infant is lacking. Based on studies of intake of breast milk in Swedish infants and the composition of human milk, the above information about average daily intake of various amino acids at different ages can be derived (Table 1.8).

Amino-acid pattern. Besides the total quantity of amino acids present, the proportion in which they occur is also important with regard to the utilisation of a protein food. The relationship of each individual amino acid to other amino acids determines the efficiency of its utilisation by the body. Hence the *pattern* of amino acids in food is one of the important factors influencing the total amount of protein required. Feeding studies in infants show that the pattern of amino acids found most suitable for supporting growth also resembles closely the pattern found in breast milk. Table 1.9 compares the patterns of requirement in infants with those of breast milk, cow's milk and egg proteins. It is obvious from the table that the protein of breast milk will be utilised with the greatest efficiency by the infant.

Table 1.9: Comparison of Patterns of Amino Acid Requirements with that of Milk and Egg Proteins (mg per g of protein)

| Amino acid | Suggested pattern of requirement[a] | Composition of protein | | |
		Human milk	Cow's milk	Egg
Histidine	14	26	27	22
Isoleucine	35	46	47	54
Leucine	80	93	95	86
Lysine	52	66	78	70
Methionine and Cystine	29	42	33	57
Phenylalanine and Tyrosine	63	72	102	93
Threonine	44	43	44	47
Tryptophan	8.5	17	14	17
Valine	47	55	64	66

[a] Joint FAO/WHO Expert Committee, 1973.

Metabolism of milk protein. Do the quality and quantity of protein in the infant's diet affect his well-being in any way? Present evidence suggests that it is almost certainly so in the case of the low birth weight infant and very likely so in the case of the normal newborn. In the

pre-term infant many of the enzyme systems in the liver are not fully
developed. For example, the mechanism for making cystine from
methionine is incomplete in the pre-term baby, so that unlike the adult
he must rely on an exogenous supply of cystine. Cow's milk is a poor
source of cystine and infants fed on cow's milk based formulae are
likely to experience a deficiency of this amino acid. In the same way,
the capacity for the *breakdown* of amino acids is impaired in pre-term
infants, especially with regard to phenylalanine and tyrosine. When
these babies are fed cow's milk based formulae, with high protein
concentrations, the blood levels of these two amino acids rise, reaching
in some cases levels as high as those in phenylketonuria. Furthermore, these high blood concentrations are known to persist for as
long as six weeks. Hence, from this point of view alone, there are
several risks in the artificial feeding of infants; these are greater in
the pre-term infant or in the infant whose physiological reserves have
been compromised by asphyxia, trauma, infection or congenital defects.

Milk Fat

The fat in milk is the main source of energy, since, per unit weight, it
provides twice the amount of energy derived from protein and sugar.

Naturally occurring fatty acids contain 4 to 24 carbon atoms in a
molecule. According to the number of carbon atoms present they are
divided into long (18 or more carbon atoms), medium (8 to 12 carbon
atoms), and short (4 to 6 carbon atoms) chain fatty acids. The short
chain fatty acids are not abundant in food fats. The medium chain acids
are also not very common, but are of interest because they are
absorbed through the portal circulation instead of the intestinal
lymphatics. Long chain fatty acids constitute the major proportion of
fat in both human and cow's milk.

The fatty acids are also classified as saturated or unsaturated,
depending upon the presence of double bonds between the carbon
atoms. The unsaturated ones may be mono- or poly-unsaturated,
depending upon the number of carbon atoms with double bonds. As a
general rule, the absorption of fatty acids in the gut is inversely related
to the number of carbon atoms. The *larger* the chain, the less
efficient is the absorption. On the other hand, the *more* the number of
double bonds the better the absorption.

In all milks the fat contains mainly long chain acids with 14 to 22
carbon atoms. Depending upon the species, the fatty acids occur in
varying quantities of saturated and unsaturated ones. An important
consideration in the synthesis of milk fat in the cow is the rumen,

which acts as a large fermentation tank with a capacity of 40 to 60 gallons, depending upon the size of the animal. Cellulose is broken down in the rumen by the action of bacteria and protozoa and the products of this fermentation, like acetate, butyrate, etc., are utilised in the synthesis of lipids. Hence cow's milk contains a large proportion of short chain fatty acids. Moreover, the lipids within the rumen, being plant lipids, are highly unsaturated when they are first released from their vegetable source. They then undergo rapid hydrogenation in the fermenting environment of the rumen and are converted into saturated fats. These are then absorbed and contribute to the saturated fatty acids of milk. In contrast, the fat in human milk consists mainly of unsaturated fatty acids.

The fatty acid composition of breast milk is dependent upon the source of fat in the mother's diet, and the total quantity of fat varies according to the adequacy of calories and other nutrients. Lipid content is also dependent upon the presence or otherwise of depot fat and its availability for the synthesis of milk fat. Thus, fatty acids of human milk are unique to each individual mother. Nonetheless one can recognise a constant pattern in the lipids of human milk. When breast milk from mothers in different countries was analysed, it was found that the most important difference lay in short chain fatty acids with 10 to 14 carbon atoms. These acids were in higher concentration in East African and Asian mothers. The high proportion of C_{10} to C_{14} acids was associated with a relatively lower proportion of C_{16} to C_{18} acids in both the saturated and unsaturated groups. This is probably due to the fact that Europeans live on a high fat diet rich in C_{16} to C_{18} acids and the mammary gland has little need to synthesise new fatty acids. The East African communities use foods which are low in fat, and the high proportion of C_{10} to C_{14} acids in their milk is due to net synthesis within the breast of fat from carbohydrate sources.

When specimens of tissue fat in infants are analysed for their fatty acid composition, it is found that the nature of body fat is largely determined by that of the dietary fat. Infants fed on human milk have a different composition of tissue fat from those fed on cow's milk or on milk formulae containing vegetable oils. This observation is important for two reasons. The brain and the rest of the nervous system undergo rapid growth throughout early infancy. Though the brain cells are largely developed by the time of birth, myelin is still to be laid along the axons and the dendritic connections. Fat is an important constituent of myelin, as indeed of the rest of the nervous system. Intake of biologically inappropriate fatty acids can produce a long-lasting effect on the growth of the nervous system. Secondly, as far as the intake of nutrients is concerned, the infant is dependent upon just one food source, the milk. Unlike the adult who eats a varied diet and has several food sources providing a rich variety of nutrients, the infant's choice is restricted to those nutrients which are present in the milk with which he is being fed. There is virtually no margin of safety and any inadequacy in the milk will be translated into altered composition of body tissues being formed at the time. Such a deficiency is then likely to be carried over to a future period when the required nutrients become available and the deficiency can be corrected. Whether such a restructuring of myelin can occur is not yet known, but present evidence suggests that it is unlikely.

In order to avoid this difficulty, the manufacturers of many brands of powdered milks modify the fat composition by removing butter fat from cow's milk and replacing it with vegetable oils. This practice gives rise to even more difficulties (Table 1.10).

Carbohydrate

Lactose is the predominant sugar in the milk of most mammals, with very few exceptions. The extremes of variation in the lactose content of the milk of mammals are from 4 g per dl in the dog and the elephant to about 7 g per dl in man. By contrast, the fat composition can vary by almost 30-fold. This relative constancy of lactose secretion in milk is an indication of its important role in mammalian biology. The nature of this role needs to be determined, but for the present one can speculate along the following lines:

(i) Amongst the various sugars, per molecule (and hence per unit of osmotic pressure) lactose provides twice the calorific value of glucose. Since milk is secreted at the same osmotic pressure as plasma, there is less energy consumed in maintaining osmotic equilibrium when lactose is used as the main sugar.

In human milk, lactose accounts for half the osmotic pressure, the remainder being due to monovalent ions like Na^+, K^+, Cl^-, etc. Because of the high concentration of lactose in breast milk, the solute content of breast milk is low, which makes it well suited for the immature kidneys of the infant.

(ii) High concentration of lactose in human milk influences the pH of the gut in the newborn and its bacterial flora. Together with other immune factors to be described below, the high lactose concentration of breast milk prevents the growth of the potentially

Table 1.10: Fatty Acid Composition of Human and Cow's Milks, Several Infant Feeding Formulae and Commonly Used Vegetable Fats in Their Manufacture

Fatty acid nomenclature	Saturated							Unsaturated				
	4:8	10:0	12:0	14:0	16:0	18:0	20:0	16:1	18:1	18:2	18:3	20:4
Human milk[a]	0.46	1.5	7.0	8.5	21.0	7.0	1.0	2.5	36.0	7.0	1.0	0.5
Cow's milk	5.5	3.0	3.5	12.0	28.0	13.0	–	3.0	28.5	1.0	–	–
SMA[b]	–	1.0	10	6	16.0	11	–	1	29.0	24.0	2.0	–
Nativa	–	2.0	9.0	9.0	22.0	7.0	–	1	35.0	13.0	1.0	–
Almiron B	–	–	–	<1	11	2	–	<1	27.0	58.0	2.0	–
Farilacid	–	2.0	2.0	9	25	14	–	2	35.0	7.0	1.0	–
Frisolac	–	<1	6.0	3.0	32.0	4.0	–	–	38.0	16.0	–	–
Similac	–	2.0	19.0	7.0	9.0	3.0	–	–	19.0	40.0	<1	–
Milumil	–	1.0	4.0	7.0	35.0	8.0	–	1	32.0	10.0	–	–
Nan	–	2.0	4.0	11.0	31.0	9.0	–	2	24.0	16.0	1	–
Humana 1 and 2	–	1.0	7.0	4.0	23.0	8.0	–	<1	44.0	13.0	<1	–
Pelargon	–	2.0	2.0	8.0	24.0	11.0	–	1.0	30.0	16.0	1	–
Oleo oils[a]	–	–	0.2	3.3	26.0	20.0	–	–	45.5	3.0	0.5	–
Corn oil	–	–	–	–	13.0	4.0	Trace	–	29.0	54.0	–	–
Coconut oil	7.0	6.0	49.5	19.5	8.5	2.0	Trace	–	6.0	1.5	–	–
Soya oil	–	–	–	Trace	11.0	4.0	Trace	–	25.0	51.0	9.0	–
Cottonseed oil	–	–	–	1.0	29.0	4.0	Trace	2.0	24.0	40.0	–	–

a Expressed as percentage by weight.   b Expressed as g/100 g total fat.

dangerous bacterium, E. coli, and instead promotes colonisation by
lactobacillus.
(iii) It is likely that lactose is utilised for the synthesis of the
galactolipids of the growing brain in the infant. In many mammalian
species the quantity of galactose per unit weight of brain tissue of
the offspring is closely related to the lactose content of the mother's
milk.
Cow's milk is low in lactose; and so, in the manufacture of many
infant feeding formulae, the first stage in the 'humanising' of cow's
milk is to increase the sugar content. This is done either by adding
more lactose or other sugars like sucrose, fructose, glucose and
dextri-maltose.

Human Milk as a Nutrient

In each mammalian species, the milk has evolved together with the
mammal to provide the offspring with nutrition best adapted to the
environment. Thus, in the whale the milk contains large amounts of fat
to help the infant lay down body fat for protection against cold and
for buoyancy. In the kangaroo, the mother has two separate nipples,
each producing milk of different composition. The new-born kangaroo
is first attached to one nipple, where he obtains milk of high protein
concentration. When the offspring is grown and can leave the pouch for
brief periods, he changes over to the other nipple and obtains from it
milk of different composition.
    The attempts of the food chemist to modify the milk of one
mammal, the cow, for feeding another, the human infant, have been
largely unsuccessful, notwithstanding the claims made in the
promotional literature. The reasons are obvious. It is not just the
question of adding a sugar to get the carbohydrate content right, or of
diluting to get the protein content right, nor of replacing butter fat
with a mixture of vegetable oils. The entire structure of the protein in
human milk is so very different from that in cow's milk (Figure 1.7).
The fatty acid composition is unique for each mother and so also are
the electrolytes and trace elements. It is not surprising that the history
of artificial feeding of infants is full of examples of one mishap after
another — starting with rickets in the early part of the century, neonatal
tetany in the early fifties, pyridoxine deficiency in the late fifties and
sixties and haemolysis due to vitamin E deficiency and risks of high
plasma sodium in more recent years. Products promoted as 'ideal
foods' are withdrawn a few years later when their shortcomings are

Figure 1.7: Comparison of the Amino Acid Pattern of Human and Cow's Milk Protein using Human Milk Protein as the Standard*

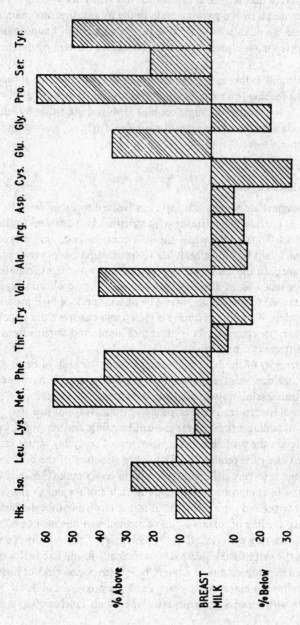

* The values, expressed as mg amino acid per g nitrogen in cow's milk, have been calculated as a percentage of those for breast milk expressed on the same basis.

Source: Food and Agriculture Organisation of the United Nations, 1970.

realised, only to be replaced by another family of products which are again promoted with equal vigour.

The uniqueness of the mother's milk in the nutrition of her infant is apparent when we consider the cellular mechanism of synthesis and secretion of its various constituents. Hormonal stimulation throughout pregnancy prepares the breasts for secretion of milk. Soon after the birth of the baby there is secretion of prolactin from the anterior pituitary. Together with other hormonal changes, it provides the stimulus for the activities of the several enzymes in the acinar cells of the mammary glands, leading to the synthesis and secretion of milk. Various cell organelles participate in the process. Synthesis occurs on the ribosomes in the rough endoplasmic reticulum in accordance with the genetic message carried within the cell nucleus. Thus, whereas the ribosomes and the rough endoplasmic reticulum provide the framework for the site of synthesis, the biological characteristics of the final product are determined by the DNA and the mRNA operating from the cell nucleus. The Golgi apparatus provides storage for the final product until it is emptied into the cell lumen. The raw materials for milk synthesis come from the mother's body either as substances circulating in the blood, e.g. amino acids, or as products stored in her tissues, e.g. fats. Ultimately they are all derived from her diet. Thus, the interaction of the genetic constitution of the mother with her environment provides the raw material for the synthesis of milk in ways determined by the genetic code in the nucleus of the alveolar cell. The infant, on the other hand, is endowed by the mother with half of his genetic make-up. Hence from the biological point of view mother's milk is most suited for the unique metabolic activity of the infant's tissues. No amount of dilution, addition, adjusting or so-called humanising of the milk of another mammal will give the characteristic configuration of molecules and biological properties of a mother's milk for her own infant.

Dangers of Artificial Feeding

We have already considered some of the dangers of feeding infants on formulae in which nutrients like proteins, fats, and carbohydrates are biologically unsuitable or present in unusual amounts. Long term epidemiological observations, as well as carefully conducted metabolic studies, would be necessary to prove such dangers in a conclusive manner. The wide range of biological variability between individuals and the physiological margins of safety, added to the adaptability of each individual make the interpretation of data difficult; there is therefore inevitable delay in obtaining conclusive evidence. For example, it has taken more than 25 years of painstaking research to prove the dangers of smoking; the relationship of saturated fats to coronary heart disease has not been conclusively established even after a similar long period of enquiry. The situation with regard to artificial feeding is similar in many ways. Thus the first reports of hypernatraemia in infants, associated with feeding of certain milk formulae, appeared in 1955, but it was not until the publication of a Working Party report in 1974 in the UK that several brands of powdered milk were withdrawn by the manufacturers. All these brands had enjoyed great popularity until then and each one had been promoted by its manufacturer as desirable for infant feeding. Yet they all contained large amounts of electrolytes, enough to tax the infant kidneys' capacity, especially in warm weather or during an episode of fever or diarrhoea (Figure 1.8). In many developing countries these brands of milk powders are still on sale. Due to the hot climate the dangers of hypernatraemia and electrolyte disturbances are even greater in the tropics.

Many of the dangers of artificial feeding arise from errors in reconstitution. In experiments in which mothers, trained midwives and health visitors took part, it was shown that there were wide individual variations in the quantity of milk powder measured for preparing a given volume of feed. The amount of milk powder measured could vary by as much as 20 to 30 per cent from that recommended by the manufacturers. In the case of babies from 'good' homes, over-concentration of feeds is the rule.

The dangers of artificial feeding are most obvious in Third World countries. Breast feeding has declined sharply in these countries in the face of intensive promotion by the manufacturers, and in the absence of a strong professional support for breast feeding. Many mothers take to artificial feeding only to find that the family income is inadequate to support the cost of powdered milk. In one survey of ten countries in the Third World it was revealed that the cost of artificial feeding a six-month-old infant could be as much as a third to a half of the minimum wage. In fact, because of the high levels of unemployment, many wage-earners accept employment at wages far lower than the statutory minimum wage. The true cost of artificial feeding could well be a sizable proportion of the family income. The temptation to 'stretch' the tin of milk powder is only too great in such a situation, with consequent underfeeding of the infant. In 1972, in Barbados, only 18 per cent of the poorer mothers were using a one pound tin of powdered milk for four days or less, as indicated by the manufacturer. The majority extended the use of the milk for five days to as much as

Figure 1.8: Urine Osmolar Load in a 5 kg Infant Fed Different Milk
Formulae at 200 ml/kg/day with Varying Insensible Loss*

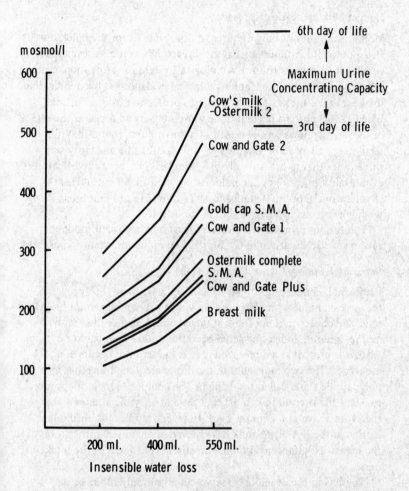

* The electrolytes in milk are eventually excreted in the infant's urine. Thus,
the higher the electrolyte content of the milk, the greater the osmolar load for
the kidney. When water loss from skin and lungs is considerable — as in hot
conditions — the urine must be concentrated and, as the figure demonstrates,
under certain conditions, this may task the kidney up to its limit.

three weeks. It is not surprising, therefore, that the decline of breast
feeding in the developing world is accompanied by a high incidence of
malnutrition in children. An additional danger in the overcrowded

homes of the poor is that of infected feeds due to lack of hygiene and the inability to care for the feeding bottles and mixing utensils properly.

Human Milk as a Protective Agent

Mother's milk is not only a source of nourishment for the baby, but also a powerful antimicrobial agent. Breast milk contains several factors which act in concert to form a biological system for protection against infection. For a long time epidemiological evidence has been indicating the benefits of breast feeding as regards protection from infection. When 1,712 mothers in rural Chile were interviewed to assess the effect of feeding practices on the health of infants, it was found that if bottle-feeding commenced before the age of 3 months, the mortality was three times that in breast-fed babies. Similarly, in the study of patterns of mortality in childhood, conducted by the Pan American Health Organisation in South America in 1973, it was found that breast feeding was a major factor in infant survival.

The various protective factors in breast milk and their modes of action are also discussed in Chapter 3. The more important factors are:

Immunoglobulins (Figure 1.9a and 1.9b)

Breast milk contains IgA, IgM, IgG and IgD. Of these, IgA occurs in the largest amounts and has been shown to play an important biological role. The concentration of IgA in breast milk is higher than in the mother's serum, indicating active secretion rather than passive transfer. Also, it is present as a dimer, whereas in the serum it occurs as a monomer. The two molecules of the dimer are joined together by a polypeptide chain called the J chain. The composite molecule is more resistant than serum IgA to pH changes and enzymic attacks and is therefore active in the infant's gut. In several studies the antibodies carried in the IgA of the milk have been demonstrated in the stools of the breast fed infant in amounts directly proportional to the intake of milk.

The IgG in breast milk also serves an important anti-infection function. It is known that during pregnancy IgG passes from the mother's blood to the infant through the placenta. Early studies on human colostrum did not show the presence of *large* amounts of IgG and it was thought that in the case of the human the only mechanism of transfer was through the placenta. However, breast fed babies have higher levels of serum IgG at 4 to 6 weeks compared to bottle-fed controls. Since the baby receives a considerable amount of IgG trans-placentally, there is presumably no urgency for large quantities to be

Figure 1.9a and b: Changes in Breast Milk Content of Lactoferrin,
Lysozyme and Immunoglobins with Duration of Lactation Measured
in 200 Women of the Lower Socio-economic Class in South India

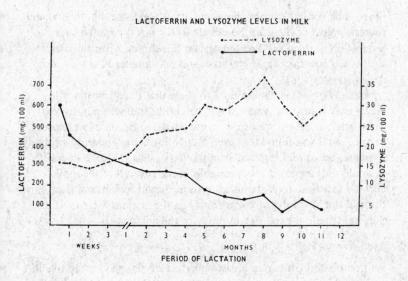

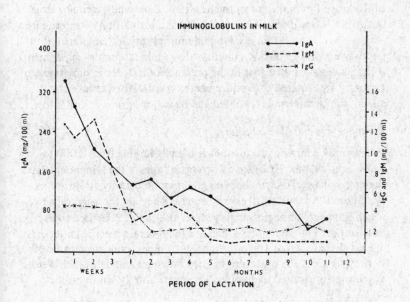

provided through the colostrum after birth, as is the case with the calf and the pig. Instead, the breast fed human infant receives IgG in small doses over a prolonged period.

Antibodies

Breast milk contains antibodies against many organisms, both viral and bacterial. Most of these antibodies are of the IgA type and a large proportion of them are directed against E. coli, though antibodies against tetanus, shigella, H. pertussis and pneumoniae have also been demonstrated.

There is experimental evidence to show that E. coli antibody in breast milk is specific against the E. coli in the mother's gut. In one experiment, pregnant women were administered E. coli of an unusual nature, and it was found that even though there was no *serum* antibody response, breast milk contained antibodies against the same E. coli. It would thus appear that plasma cells in the gut wall of the mother become sensitised to bacterial antigens in the gut lumen, and then move through the blood stream to 'home in' on the mammary gland where they contribute the specific antibody to the milk.

Lactoferrin (Figure 1.9b).

An iron-binding protein in breast milk, lactoferrin, plays a key role in the action of IgA on the bacterium E. coli by inhibiting the proliferation of this organism in the gut of the newborn. Breast milk contains large quantities of lactoferrin – 2-6 mg/ml. It has a high affinity for ferric iron which E. coli requires for growth and multiplication. Lactoferrin thus deprives E. coli of iron and growth is slowed. In laboratory experiments it can be demonstrated that in the presence of lactoferrin only traces of antibody are required to produce bacteriostasis. When excess iron is added, the lactoferrin is saturated and its action against E. coli is lost.

Lymphocytes and Macrophages

Human milk contains a large number of cells varying from 2,000 to 4,000 cells/cu mm. These are of two main types – the lymphocyte and the macrophage. The lymphocytes are immunologically active and synthesise IgA as well as β1c complement. They are the same cells which 'home in' on the mammary gland after being sensitised to bacterial antigens in the mother's gut, and they secrete specific antibodies against these bacteria. The macrophages of breast milk are capable of destroying klebsiella organisms in vitro. In animal models which were appropriately stressed by hypoxia they were also shown to protect against necrotising enterocolitis.

Other Factors

Breast milk contains large amounts of the C_3 and C_4 components of complement, which can be activated in experimental conditions by the antibody contained in the IgA of the milk. It also contains lysozyme in large amounts, averaging up to 29-39 mg/100 ml. The exact mechanism of action of these substances has not yet been fully determined. It has been postulated that they interact together as a biological system in mounting immunological attacks on bacteria in the baby's gut.

In addition there is the bifidus factor which promotes the growth of the lactobacillus organism under the specific pH and chemical environment of the neonatal gut generated by breast milk. The gut flora of the artificially-fed infant is made up largely of E. coli, with some Streptococcus faecalis, in contrast to the breast-fed infant in whom the lactobacillus predominates. The E. coli harboured by the gut of the artificially-fed infant constitute a reservoir of potential pathogens. The exact conditions under which they can cause disease are not yet understood. The immune factors in breast milk will keep the number of E. coli in the gut low until such time as the baby has developed his own immunity. In this way breast milk is unique. It is an agent which protects at the same time as it nourishes and the mammary gland performs a function not very different from that of the placenta in intrauterine life.

Closely related to protection from infection is the role of human milk in preventing hypersensitivity. Secretory IgA in the gut lumen is known to prevent the adsorption of antigen on the gut mucosa. When there is a deficiency of IgA, macromolecules of antigen in the gut lumen are able to pass through the mucosal cells and enter the blood stream or lymphatics and trigger an immune response. Breast milk, with its high content of IgA, prevents the escape of antigen into the blood stream and thus protects against atopic disease (see Chapter 3).

Mother-Infant Relationship

The act of suckling is a form of intimate communication between the mother and her infant, and it contributes to the creation of the love bond between the two. The skin contact, the eye-to-eye or 'en face' position adopted during or soon after feeding, the satisfaction of hunger in the infant and the pleasurable tactile stimulation in the mother during suckling all promote the process of bonding between the two. In many mammals, the time of birth is a critical period during which imprinting occurs, so that the mother recognises her offspring and vice versa. Similar imprinting during a critical period also occurs in the human, and breast feeding plays an important role in this process. Mothers who are separated from their infants, for medical or other reasons, at this critical period, have a higher incidence of rejection of their babies and of child abuse.

The Weaning Period

Most infants thrive well on their mother's milk alone in the first three to four months of life. This is a period of rapid growth. The average infant is expected to increase his birth weight by more than half and grow in length by ten per cent during this time. The demands for nutrients are higher than at any time in life. It is estimated that the normal two or three-month-old infant is likely to consume 116 kcal/kg/day and probably absorbs more than 100 kcal/kg/day. By contrast, a 70 kg young adult male will rarely absorb as much as 50 kcal/kg/day. Thus the infant's digestive tract is more remarkable for its high capacity for absorption than for any limitations; it is functioning close to capacity in order to keep up with the demands of rapid growth. Approximately one-third of the energy intake between birth and the age of four months may be accounted for by synthesis of new tissues. By contrast, during the growth spurt of puberty, which is another period of rapid growth, the adolescent utilises less than 10 per cent of his energy intake for growth, even during periods of peak growth.

It is remarkable that breast milk alone can supply all the nutrients necessary to support such rapid growth. Studies on growth of infants in Gambia, Uganda and Guatemala have shown that in many instances the rate of growth may even be greater than that of English or American infants of the same age. The output of breast milk keeps pace with demand until about the age of 3-4 months when it reaches the maximum and cannot increase further. It is at this time that the growth of a large proportion of children in the developing world begins to slow down. Thus in Uganda it was found that there is a sharp fall in the velocity of weight gain between the ages of three and six months, and a further fall between six and nine months to a rate of only half of that in English children. After the age of nine months the velocity of weight gain gradually improves, but continues to be lower than that of English children until the age of eighteen months. The rates of weight gain in the second and third years of life are similar to those of English children, but the ground lost in the early period is never made up. Growth in height also suffers in the same way. There is a sharp fall in the rate of increase in length from the age of three months, so that at six months the velocity of growth in height is less than 85 per cent of that of English children. It begins to improve at the age of one year and reaches the normal rate at about 1½ years, after which it continues at the normal rate in the second and third years. Again the ground lost in the early period is not recovered. Thus growth in both weight and height is most severely affected between three and 12 months of age, and the slowing of growth in the first year of life accounts for 91 per cent of the deficit in body weight and 98 per cent of the deficit in length at the age of three. Such a faltering of growth in the first year of life is characteristic of the majority of children in the Third World. Though their rate of growth approaches the standard in the second and third years, when growth is normally slowing down, the lost ground is never recovered and the deficit remains.

Dangers of the Weaning Period

The weaning period is fraught with danger for a large proportion of the world's children and nutritional disorders are common at this time of life. In the West a general awareness of the nutritional needs of the weanling, together with the ability of the average family to provide the necessary foods, have helped to remove most of the dangers of the weaning period. In the peasant society, however, parents are generally unaware of the dietary needs of children, and several customs associated with weaning are likely to give rise to nutritional deficiencies. For example, in many parts of India the ceremony of 'Anna Prasanna' must be carried out at the time of weaning. In this ceremony, several kinds of foods are cooked and offered to the deity to invoke her blessings. Family and kinsmen are entertained during the celebrations. Often weaning is delayed until such time as the family have been able to save for the expense of the ceremony. In Uganda and among several communities along the shores of Lake Victoria, the common practice is to separate the child from his mother in order to take him off the breast and to get him to eat other foods. The weanling is sent away to live with the grandparents for a few months. The unhappiness of separation is added to the nutritional upset caused by a sudden change from a highly nutritious food to a gruel.

In the traditional society weaning is commonly abrupt and unplanned. Often it is brought about by the occurrence of another pregnancy in the mother. In many communities there are superstitions and beliefs concerning the effects of another pregnancy on the quality of breast milk. It is believed that the heat from the womb 'poisons' the breast milk. Also that the baby in the womb is jealous of the older sibling on the breast. It is therefore considered urgent that the child should be taken off the breast immediately. In the ensuing hurry, there is hardly any time for the gradual introduction of solids to allow the child to get used to them. Instead, the breast is denied to him. The mother may apply potions to her nipples so that when the child takes the breast, their sharp bitter taste makes him give up suckling. The practice of separating the mother from the child is yet another way of effecting abrupt weaning.

By the age of 6 months, weaning has commenced in most children with small supplements prepared out of local foods. Commonly it is a gruel or pap made from the local staple. Here again, traditional practices, advice from the elders or family members, and the mother's own experience determines the type and consistency of the weaning diet (Figure 1.10).

Figure 1.10: Determinants of Weaning Practices

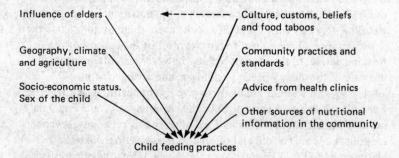

Child feeding practices

Traditional Dietary Practices

In the traditional dietary breast milk provides the foundation to which other weaning foods can be gradually added. In a field study in Uganda it was noticed that during their second year breast-fed infants obtained 91 kcal/kg body weight and the non-breast-fed infants consumed 68 kcal/kg body weight per day. After breast feeding was stopped the intake of other foods was increased by 60 per cent, but it was still not sufficient to make up for the energy supplied by the breast milk. The reason is that human milk has a relatively high energy density at 6 kcal/g dry matter and the transition to a diet of relatively low energy density is the cause of many nutritional problems. This concept of 'energy density' of the diet is an important advance in our knowledge of weaning foods.

Studies of food intake in young children from several countries confirm the above findings. In all peasant communities, energy intake with the traditional weaning foods is well below requirements. The intake of energy becomes inadequate soon after the third month and does not increase much between the ages of seven and thirty months. Protein intake, though low, increases with age. The current view is that inadequate intake of energy, and not of protein, is the main aetiological factor in infantile malnutrition.

At first glance it may appear that the intake of energy could be increased by increasing the number of feeds offered to the child. In practice, however, this is not so simple. For example the field study on Ugandan children showed that children fed *ad libitum* five times daily consumed the same energy as those fed three times. With the traditional diet, the capacity for intake was in the range of 90-95 kcal/kg body weight daily. When food was offered less frequently at home it was not possible to achieve this level of intake. Increasing the energy content with fats and edible oils would be one way of improving the intake of energy without affecting the capacity for intake.

Food Intake and Appetite in the Weanling

When daily food intakes in infants and young children are monitored over a period of time, the important role of appetite in the control of food intake becomes clear. In the study of Ugandan infants, it was found that, below the age of six months, less than 10 per cent of children suffered from anorexia, but after that age lack of appetite was reported in 25 to 40 per cent by their mothers. The highest prevalence of poor appetite was in the age group between 13 and 18 months. Anorexia was often due to illness, the frequency of which rose sharply after the age of six months. The prevalence of anorexia can be appreciated from the fact that between the age of 7 and 24 months, the average Ugandan child did not eat well on 1 day out of 3, and from the third year onwards on 1 day out of 4.

Even when the child ate well, the traditional bulky food provided not more than 100 kcal/kg body weight daily. Such an intake is just enough for normal weight gain and for maintenance of serum albumin levels, but not for catch-up growth after an illness. If the energy density of the traditional food were to be raised from 100-125 kcal/100 g to

125-150 kcal/100 g by the means mentioned, the energy intake of a
10 kg child would be increased by 250 kcal per day. This increased
energy intake will provide a small margin of safety for such periods when
food intake is diminished by anorexia. Again, the importance of breast
milk in the second year of life is well demonstrated by this study. By
providing additional energy and protein it helps to offset the energy
constraints of the traditional weaning foods. The mean daily intake of
energy in infants who were not breast fed was barely adequate for
maintenance even with a good appetite. Although the intake of protein
was more than the requirement, much of the protein was utilised for
energy and, as such, wasted.

To summarise, the traditional weaning foods, together with episodes
of anorexia caused by illnesses, lead to restricted energy intake in the
first year of life. After that, in the second year, the transition from a
diet with a relatively high energy concentration, viz. breast milk, to one
with low energy concentration leads to intakes of energy which are
only just about at maintenance levels for a considerable period of time.

The Role of Intercurrent Infections

Infections and intercurrent illnesses play an important role in the
aetiology of nutritional disorders. The episodes of illness increase after
the age of six months as the passive immunity derived from the
mother begins to decline. The common infectious diseases of childhood,
like chickenpox, whooping cough, measles, etc. usually occur in the
first 3 or 4 years of life. Respiratory infections and, in endemic areas,
episodes of malaria occur repeatedly after the first 4 months. Diarrhoea
is also common and a well-recognised hazard of the weaning period, as
indicated by the phrase 'weanling diarrhoea'. Diarrhoeal episodes at
the time of weaning are common in several mammals, like the cat and
the pig, and in both they are known to be lethal. Several explanations
have been put forth to account for weanling diarrhoea. Irritation of the
gut by new and unaccustomed foods, change from a liquid to a semi-
solid diet and many other factors have been mentioned. But above all,
ingestion of contaminants and large numbers of pathogens would appear
to be the most important cause according to recent studies in Gambia.

Each episode of infection causes a slowing of growth and even loss
of weight if the illness has been severe (Figure 1.11). This is followed by
a period of catch-up growth during recovery. If the interval between
infections is too short, catch-up growth cannot occur and there is
progressive deterioration in the nutritional status. Again the amount of
bulk in the diet is an important consideration. If the food contains as

Figure 1.11: Catch-up
Growth in Two Children*

See also p. 76

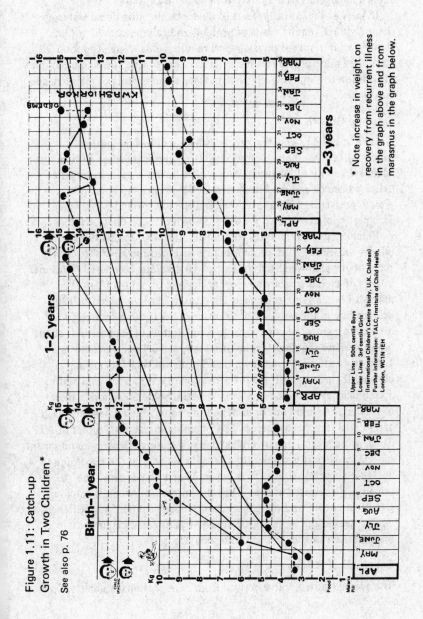

* Note increase in weight on
recovery from recurrent illness
in the graph above and from
marasmus in the graph below.

Upper Line: 50th centile Boys
Lower Line: 3rd centile Girls
(International Children's Centre Study, U.K. Children)
Further information: TALC, Institute of Child Health,
London, WC1N 1EH

as 1 kcal/g a child weighing 10 kg would need to eat 1 kg of the
daily to consume enough calories. A sick child who is anorexic,
coughing or vomiting would need to consume 300 to 500 g of the food
at each meal and this may well be beyond his capacity.

In view of the known effects of illness on the nutritional status of
the individual, requirements of proteins and calories should not be
thought of in terms of physiological requirements alone. The food
consumed must provide a substantial cushion for the stress of infection
in addition to supplying the physiological requirements of maintenance
and growth.

Catch-up Growth

Growth is a highly sensitive process which requires the optimal
functioning of the body's physiological processes together with an
adequate supply of nutrients. Any illness, however mild, upsets the
delicate balance and growth falters. Under normal circumstances,
growth accelerates during recovery and the lost ground is recovered.
This period of accelerated growth is known as catch-up growth.

Catch-up growth requires additional nutrients. Observations on
infants recovering from protein-calorie malnutrition have shown that
such infants gain weight at the rate of 10 g/kg/day compared to normal
infants of the same size who grow at the rate of 3.3 g/kg/day. The
malnourished infants consumed 169 kcal/kg/day compared to 120
kcal/kg/day in the normals. Thus, assuming that the increased food
intake represents the cost of tissue formed, it would appear that about
50-80 kcal are required for the formation of 10 g body weight.
Laboratory studies have shown that 3 moles of ATP (adenosine tri-
phosphate) are required for the activation of each amino acid and its
attachment by a peptide bond to a protein. Some 6 or more moles
of ATP may be used up for each peptide bond which is formed. Each
amino acid transported across a cell membrane uses up 3 moles of ATP.
Thus, protein synthesis is very expensive in terms of energy requirement,
especially when it is realised that for glucose and fat the maximum
energy convertible to ATP is between 38 and 40 per cent. The
remainder is released as heat. Thus the nutritional needs of catch-up
growth are heavy and there is a need for concentrated forms of energy
and protein in the weanling's diet. The traditional diets, in most
instances, are unable to cope with such needs.

Longitudinal Studies

The average growth curve derived from cross-sectional studies or from annual measurements of a cohort of children conceals cycles of growth impairment caused by seasonal falls in food supply or illnesses. Studies have therefore been undertaken in which accurate measurements were made of daily food intake of young children over a period of time, maintaining records of illnesses and observing the effects of both on the growth of children. Such studies have been reported from India, Guatemala, Uganda and Gambia. Together they have thrown further light on the interaction of causative factors in childhood malnutrition. Until recently it was thought that the two clinical syndromes of kwashiorkor and marasmus stemmed from different types of nutritional deficiency. It was believed that kwashiorkor was mainly due to deficiency of protein and that marasmus was caused by inadequate intake of calories. Creation of laboratory models of the two syndromes in animals by the restriction of proteins or total calories gave further support to such hypotheses. Several international meetings under the aegis of UN agencies discussed 'the world protein gap' and explored the possibilities of increasing the production of protein foods. Data from the longitudinal studies mentioned have helped to rectify some of the wrong concepts regarding infantile malnutrition.

Studies carried out by the National Institute of Nutrition in Hyderabad, India, provided the first evidence on the basis of which the above view was questioned. Three hundred children were observed from birth onwards for varying periods and 90 of them until the age of 3 years. It was found that growth was satisfactory up to the age of 4 months, after which growth curves flattened and there were varying degrees of emaciation. In some it was sufficiently severe to be labelled marasmus. Seven children developed frank kwashiorkor. Analysis of the dietary patterns in these children revealed that there was no difference in types and quantities of food consumed between children who developed kwashiorkor and those who did not. Similarly, there was no qualitative difference in the foods consumed and in the protein:calorie ratio of the diets between cases of kwashiorkor and marasmus or between cases of clinical malnutrition on the one hand and the other growth retarded children in the community on the other. It was obvious that cases of kwashiorkor and marasmus were the end results of more severe degrees of the same type of protein-calorie deficiency prevalent in the rest of the community. Another revealing observation was that 5 of 7 children who developed kwashiorkor had suffered recurrent bouts of diarrhoea for some days, during which appetite had been lost and food intake reduced. These children were fed their usual foods, but in smaller quantities. In one child

chickenpox had preceded kwashiorkor. In one child the onset
of kwashiorkor was gradual, with no special precipitating factors.
On the basis of their study, the Hyderabad researchers came to the
conclusion that during nutritional deficiency the growth of the child
slows to adapt to the low intake of nutrients. They further suggested
that a breakdown in the physiological process of adaptation produces
the clinical picture of kwashiorkor and that the stress of infection is a
common cause of such a failure of adaptation. This view gains further
support from similar observations made elsewhere.

The results of the Indian study are similar to those reported from
Uganda and mentioned earlier. Investigators at the Infantile
Malnutrition Unit in Kampala studied 40 children in a rural area from
birth to the age of three. The daily intakes of energy and protein were
measured and records of illnesses were maintained. Their findings
regarding the important role of breast milk in the second year of life,
that of calorie density, and the effects of anorexia caused by illness
have already been mentioned. Their work emphasised the frequency of
illness episodes during the weaning period in many developing
countries (Table 1.11).

Table 1.11: Total Number of Illnesses Per Hundred Children

	Kampala	Newcastle
Upper respiratory tract infections	74	13
Lower respiratory tract infections	258	124
Diarrhoea	107	20
Skin sepsis	160	8
Measles	36	18
Round worms	33	—
Hook worms	48	—
Malaria	257	—

From this table it is apparent that recurrent illnesses and their
influence on appetite may be more important in childhood malnutrition
than nutritional deficiency by itself.

The role of measles in the aetiology of malnutrition in tropical
Africa has been described by Morley in Nigeria. It is not unusual for a
child to lose up to 5 per cent of his body weight in a severe attack of
measles, especially when there was a weight deficit to begin with. These
early observations have now been confirmed by other workers.

Traditional beliefs about the aetiology of the disease and food taboos related to it make measles one of the commonest precipitating factors in childhood malnutrition in many parts of the Third World.

More recently, studies on the ecology of malnutrition in Gambia have shown that diarrhoeal disease may well be as important as measles, if not more. The Gambian workers found that between the ages of 7 to 13 months, children in the study villages suffered from diarrhoea for six days in each month. Unlike measles, which is an acute illness, diarrhoea is recurrent and the adverse effects of several episodes of diarrhoea tend to be cumulative. In Gambia, diarrhoea was found to be almost exclusively the non-dietary element in failure to grow. Bacteriological examination of wells and household water pots showed heavy contamination with faecal coliforms, the average bacterial count being 1,600 per 100 ml of water. Considering that water with coliform counts in excess of 10 per 100 ml is usually considered unsuitable for drinking, the above counts indicate the extent of contamination. Naturally, this was also reflected in the gruels and other foods used for feeding infants. Freshly cooked food was generally acceptable in quality, but on keeping for half an hour unacceptable levels of pathogens could be detected in the foods. When children with a history of protracted diarrhoea were studied for the bacteriology of the upper bowel, 76 per cent showed bacterial counts of 10^4 per ml compared to the upper levels of normal at 10^3. The spectrum of organisms found was also different from the normal bowel flora.

Very similar results were obtained in Guatemala, where a cohort of 45 village children were the subject of a longitudinal study, including the prevalence of diarrhoea. The peak prevalence of diarrhoea was 87 per 100 person-months in the age group 18 to 23 months. Contamination of water and food was an important element in the transmission of diarrhoeal illness. Bacterial counts in tortillas, the common staple food, were suppressed by cooking only temporarily. Within hours they became alarmingly high. Among the illnesses causing loss of weight, diarrhoea, measles and whooping cough produced maximum damage, especially in children who were already underweight. In such children an episode of one of these illnesses could lead to a weight loss of as much as 5 per cent.

The information obtained from the various studies described above has helped to challenge the orthodox view of the aetiology of malnutrition in several ways. It is now widely accepted that in the traditional dietaries the overriding deficiency is that of calories. Whenever the diets were judged to be low in protein, they were so because the *total* food intake was low. Much of the protein is then burnt to provide energy instead of being utilised as protein. The implication is that had the children consumed a sufficient amount of their usual food to provide the energy requirement, they would have consumed enough proteins also.

Secondly, it is now realised that in the past too much emphasis has been put on protein, especially on that of *animal* origin. True, protein is essential, but only like all other essential nutrients. For example, fat-soluble vitamins are essential and deficiency disorders arise when they are not consumed in adequate quantities. But in excess they cause toxic symptoms. Water-soluble vitamins are equally essential. When large quantities are ingested, the body excretes them because, unlike fat-soluble vitamins, a mechanism for excretion exists. In the same way protein is essential, but when consumed in excess the body burns it as calories and excess protein is disposed of. It is of course an uneconomical way of obtaining calories, both financially and biochemically. The yield of ATP from protein is in the range of 32 to 34 per cent compared to 38 to 40 per cent with carbohydrates and fats. This change in the status of protein from its exalted position in the past and the events leading to such re-thinking have been well described by McLaren as 'The great protein fiasco'.

Thirdly, the contribution of infection to malnutrition has hitherto been underestimated. The reasons are obvious. The observed inadequacies of traditional weaning foods, the clinical response to feeding in patients suffering from malnutrition, the creation of laboratory models of kwashiorkor and marasmus, have all helped to generate the view that nutritious food was the only thing that mattered. The above studies from different parts of the world show that the origin of malnutrition rests in two factors: (i) the lack of adequate technology at the level of the village home for preparing adequate weaning foods and (ii) lack of knowledge for avoiding the microbial pathogens in the environment.

The Role of Infection in the Aetiology of Malnutrition

As already noted, the energy cost of protein synthesis is high. Up to 15 moles of ATP, and possibly more, are used up per each amino acid in the synthesis of tissue proteins. An adult synthesising 400 g of protein per day for the normal protein turnover requires 1.4 kcal/g protein or 600 kcal for the purpose. In malnourished children the daily protein turnover is in the range of 15 to 18 g/kg body weight during the phase of recovery. This amount of protein represents a large quantity of energy, which thus becomes an important constraint in protein synthesis.

During infective illnesses, complex changes occur in protein metabolism. There is an increased flux of amino acids from skeletal muscle; phenylalanine, tryptophan, alanine and glutamine move into the extra-cellular compartment, mainly as a result of increased catabolism in the skeletal muscles, and perhaps also in skin protein. The synthesis of visceral proteins in heart and brain is not significantly affected. Also the synthesis of intrahepatic proteins is not altered, but amino acids are utilised at an accelerated rate by the liver for the synthesis of acute phase plasma globulins and for conversion to carbohydrate (gluco-neogenesis). Amino acids are also utilised by leucocytes for the synthesis of antibody, gamma-globulin and other factors involved in the immune mechanisms. The caloric needs of the body are also increased under the stress of infection, but because of the accompanying anorexia the consumption of calories is low. The septic patient is unable to mobilise his fat stores or synthesise ketones at a rate fast enough to meet his calorie needs. The result is a marked increase in gluconeogenesis from amino acids and an increased breakdown of skeletal muscle to supply these substrates. It is not surprising therefore that the negative nitrogen balance during severe infection can be four times that during starvation. For example, in starvation 4 g of nitrogen are excreted daily in urine, whereas in the septic patient nitrogen excretion may be as much as 15 g/day. As the wasting of body protein continues, the short supply of certain amino acids, such as the branched chain amino acids, can be rate limiting. This in turn causes a depletion of host proteins and a reduction in the body's defence mechanisms. Children with clinical malnutrition simply do not have sufficient nutritional stores to effect the metabolic responses like those described above in well-nourished adults during acute infections. Similar metabolic responses also occur after elective surgery or injury. In adult patients admitted to hospital for elective surgery weight loss equivalent to between 6 and 8 per cent of body weight is not unusual. A general increase in the resting metabolic expenditure of 10 to 30 per cent above basal has been described after multiple fractures and increases of 25 to 45 per cent after sepsis and 40 to 100 per cent after major burns. This increase in the resting metabolic expenditure represents an erosion of body tissues in response to injury or infection and must be recovered from a nourishing diet during convalescence.

Catabolic responses occur in all infectious illnesses regardless of the microbial agent or the presence of symptoms. Even subclinical or silent infections induce stress responses with increased nitrogen excretion in the urine, though naturally the intensity of catabolic response is proportional to the severity of the illness. As a result of such responses the energy requirements of the body are increased and skeletal muscle is catabolised to provide the substrate for energy.

The metabolic changes during infection are of three types: (i) over-utilisation of nutrients (ii) sequestration of nutrients and (iii) diversion of nutrients. In over-utilisation there is increased expenditure of energy sources like glycogen, mobilisation of amino acids for gluco-neogenesis, mobilisation of fat and over-utilisation of vitamins. Sequestration of iron in the liver explains the anaemia of children who have suffered recurrent infections. Nutrient diversion occurs when plasma amino acids are utilised for the synthesis of acute phase reactant proteins.

Gut Dynamics in Malnutrition

As we have noted earlier, the gut is working at full capacity during infancy in order to absorb the nutrients required for the rapid growth during that period. Any adverse influences on gut dynamics will affect digestion and absorption of nutrients and will interfere with growth. The epithelial cells of the small intestine are highly differentiated both morphologically and biochemically to carry out the processes of digestion, absorption and transport. These cells, or enterocytes, begin their life cycle in the crypts of the villi and travel to reach the tip as they mature. They are finally sloughed in the gut lumen at the end of their life cycle, which normally lasts from 2 to 5 days.

In the disease kwashiorkor, there is extensive damage to the mucosa of the gut. At the same time there is a reduction in the secretions of the digestive enzymes, notably the secretions of the pancreas. Various forms of malabsorption occur in keeping with these changes. In marasmus, the mucosal structure is generally normal on light microscopy, though various intracellular changes can be seen with the electron microscope. Gut function in children who are marginally undernourished has not been studied extensively. No gross defects in absorption have yet been described in such children. On the other hand, morphological changes in gut mucosa are known to occur in healthy individuals living in a tropical environment. These changes have been described both in the indigenous populations as well as in expatriates living in the tropics. In the latter, the morphological changes are known to revert to normal on return to the home environment. Whether this so-called 'tropical intestine', characterised by stunting of villi and other changes in mucosal architecture, is due to dietary factors or is caused by recurrent non-specific microbial insults is not known. Its incidence and its effects on the absorptive capacity of the gut have also not been fully studied.

Alteration of the gut flora in established cases of malnutrition has been desribed in several countries. Whether such an alteration of gut flora also occurs in marginally nourished children living in a contaminated environment is not known. Similarly, little is known about the effects of diarrhoeal disease on the absorption and utilisation of nutrients. Preliminary studies in Guatemala indicate that moderate diarrhoea may result in an increased loss of calories in the stool to the extent of 500 to 600 calories per day.

Intervention Programmes

Until recently most intervention programmes were based on the free issue of food supplements, chiefly dried skimmed milk powder either by itself or as a 'mix' with other foods. The presence of large surpluses of defatted milk in the West has led to its dumping in the hungry parts of the world under the guise of 'aid'. In many instances the thriving agribusiness in the Western world has lobbied government departments to make sure that conditions attached to the aid programme help to create new markets for their products in the Third World. Food aid has been often used as a lever by donor countries to influence policies and decisions of governments in the Third World. As far as peasant societies are concerned, however, free hand-outs have only given rise to dependency and taken away local initiative.

The whole aspect of intervention at village level is now being reassessed in many countries and several alternative approaches are being developed, aimed at improving knowledge and skills at village level for the production of appropriate weaning foods.

Multimixes

Most rural diets tend to be monotonous and are based on the local staple which is the chief source for satisfying hunger. Vegetables, legumes, and occasionally animal foods are used as relishes and to improve the palatability of the diet. The amount of relish consumed depends partly on its availability and partly on custom. As we have seen, this diet is not always adequate to meet the requirements of the weaning period. Recent trends in nutrition science emphasise the use of food mixtures in correct proportions in order to provide a balanced diet. The object is to use multimixes in such a way that up to 7 or 8 per cent of total calories are derived from net utilisable protein. I have described this concept of net dietary protein calories per cent (NdpCal per cent) elsewhere (Ebrahim, 1975) and methods of calculating the amounts of foods to be used as multimixes have been developed. Based on these principles, multimixes from locally available foods have been recommended for different regions of the Third World. If the multimix is consumed in amounts sufficient to provide the daily requirement of calories, then the requirement of protein and other nutrients will be largely taken care of.

This concept is useful not only for the education of the individual parent but also for promoting community *feeding* programmes.

The Question of Bulk in the Weaning Diet

The staple foods as well as sources of vegetable protein have a large cellulose and fibre content, which increases their bulk. A child has to consume large quantities of the multimix to obtain his daily requirements and, as we have seen, during periods of anorexia his capacity for eating may be limited. Hence it is necessary to consider ways and means of increasing the calorie *density* of the weaning food, especially during illness. Fats and oils are the obvious sources of calories, but the traditional foods of many peasant societies do not use much fat in cooking. Exceptions occur in West Africa, where the red palm oil is used in cooking and in coastal or island communities, where the use of coconut or its oil is common. In all other situations, the use of edible oils like cottonseed oil, sunflower oil, or foods with high fat content, like ground nuts, soya beans or sesame seeds, needs to be promoted in the preparation of weaning foods. For example, a double mix made from 100 g of maize flour and 25 g of legume has an NdpCal of between 7 and 8 per cent. A one-year-old child has a calorie requirement of 1180 kcalories and must eat 330 g of the mix daily. Allowing for the absorption of water during cooking, the total weight of the cooked product which must be consumed will be in the region of 550 g. If 2 teaspoons of cooking oil were used, the quantities required to give the same NdpCal per cent will be 50 g maize, 10 g oil and 25 g legume (Figure 1.12). To obtain the daily requirement the

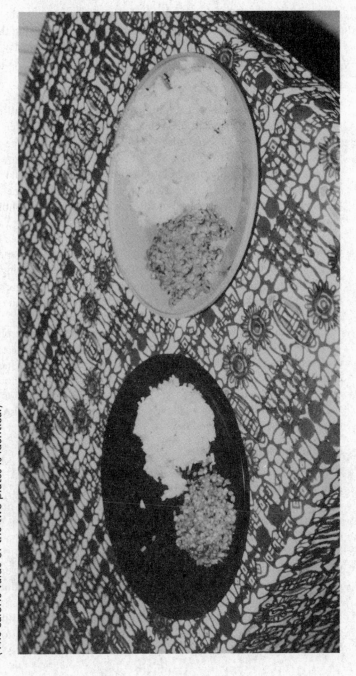

Figure 1.12: Bulk in the Diet — Double-mix Rice and Legume with and without the addition of 10 g oil. (The calorie value of the two plates is identical)

child needs to eat 375 g of the cooked product daily, which is well within his capability. By comparison, the average one-year-old in the West, eating a commercial 'junior' food, must eat 500 g in one day with 15 oz milk to obtain his daily requirements.

Prevention of Contamination

The problem of microbial contamination of food and water is a difficult one. Its solution is dependent upon the availability of a safe water supply, improvement of standards of cleanliness, personal hygiene and protection of the food from flies. Several studies have noted that bacterial counts in freshly prepared foods are of an acceptable nature, but rise quickly on keeping. At certain times of the year, as in the planting or harvesting seasons, all members of the peasant household must work long hours and the care of the weanling is delegated to an elderly relative or to a sibling. The child is fed on the food cooked by the mother before going to work and kept for several hours. Inevitably it gets contaminated and the incidence of diarrhoea tends to be high during these seasons. Provision of community creches and playgroups where freshly cooked food is offered to the children would be one way of avoiding contamination of food in the village.

Early management of diarrhoea with oral glucose-electrolyte solution in the home will prevent the development of serious dehydration or protracted diarrhoea. Like the concept of Ndpcal per cent, the glucose-electrolyte solution has helped to take the management of diarrhoea into the village home. Early recovery will prevent the deterioration of the child's general nutrition which usually happens when the episode of diarrhoea drags on for several days.

Provision of Health Services

Regular health surveillance of the children to identify those at risk will help to identify those families who need advice and help. In many Western countries infant mortality began to decline appreciably only after the large scale introduction of the infant welfare movement. Many of the important principles of the national infant welfare clinic have been adapted to the needs of rural children in the development of the under-fives' clinic. Such clinics are a useful way of combining several forms of intervention. Growth supervision, immunisation, nutrition education, treatment of minor ailments, home visiting and identification of those 'at risk' are all combined into one service programme with far-reaching impact on the health of children. Community participation in the several functions of the under-fives' clinic also helps to interest and involve the community in the health of its children.

Part-time Village Health Workers

Many of the functions of advising parents with regard to multimixes, carrying out regular health surveillance of village children, providing emergency treatment and first aid during acute emergencies, can be well performed by the part-time village health worker. In several projects such a worker has been shown to be successful in raising community awareness of the needs of children and other vulnerable groups. Since such workers are normally selected by the community and are long-time residents of the village, they also act as useful links between health services and the community. The part-time village health worker has an important contribution to make in improving the health and nutrition of village children through intervention at the level of the village home.

Protein-Energy Malnutrition

Protein-energy malnutrition (PEM) is currently the most widespread and serious health problem of children in the world, for at any time approximately 100 million children suffer from the moderate or severe forms of PEM. In any one country the number of children suffering from the disorder will be influenced by the season, the availability of food, the prevalence of infection and other such factors. As can be expected, the peak of incidence is immediately after epidemics of infectious illnesses and diarrhoea, or in the 'hungry' months. Results of community surveys during the past 10 years in 17 different countries and involving 175,000 children reveal an aggregate prevalence rate of 20 per cent (Table 1.12).

Taking the median values, an approximation of the geographical distribution of childhood malnutrition can be made in Table 1.13. The figures in Table 1.13 provide only an estimate of the size of the problem. Exact statistics will not become available until health services of the developing countries are able to achieve universal coverage of the population and efficient methods for the collection of health data are established. At present only 20 per cent of rural populations receive health care on a regular basis and most health statistics are rudimentary. Thus community surveys at regular intervals provide the only means of measuring the size of the problem. As a result of such surveys it is possible to generalise that at any time 10 per

Table 1.12: The Prevalence of Childhood Malnutrition

Area	No. of surveys	No. of children examined (,000)	Severe forms Range (%)	Severe forms Median (%)	Moderate forms Range (%)	Moderate forms Median (%)
Latin America	11	109	0.5– 6.3	1.6	3.5–32.0	18.9
Africa	7	25	1.7– 9.8	4.4	5.4–44.9	26.5
Asia	7	39	1.1–20.0	3.2	16.0–46.4	31.2
Total	25	173	0.5–20.0	2.6	3.5–46.4	18.9

Table 1.13: Geographical Distribution of Childhood Malnutrition

Area	Population aged 0–5 years (millions)	No. of children with PEM (millions) Severe	No. of children with PEM (millions) Moderate
South America	46	0.7	8.8
Africa	61	2.7	16.3
Asia	206	6.6	64.4
Total	313	10.0	89.5

cent of the children in an average peasant community will show signs of growth failure and some of them will have clinical signs of malnutrition. Only 24 per cent of children in such communities show adequate growth and the remaining 66 per cent experience faltering of growth from time to time.

The level of preschool mortality in a country may also indicate the prevalence of childhood malnutrition. This is because of the well-known synergism between nutrition and infection. The preschool mortality in the average developing country is about 40 times that of western countries, which again reveals the size of the problem. Recently, in a study of the patterns of childhood mortality in 13 areas in South America, sponsored by the Pan American Health Organisation, 7,318 deaths in children between the ages of 1-4 years were studied. Malnutrition was found to be the primary cause of death in 9 per cent (range 0-18 per cent) and an associated cause of death in 48.4 per cent (range 0 to 61 per cent). The general conclusion was that malnutrition was directly or indirectly responsible for 57.4 per cent of deaths of children aged 1-4 years.

Classification and Definition

It is paradoxical that such a widespread, serious and extensively studied
form of nutritional disorder still continues to be a controversial subject
in almost every aspect. This is especially so with regard to
classification and pathogenesis. The reason is that the presenting
features of nutritional deficiency vary from one part of the world to
another, due mainly to the great variation in the nutrient content of the
diet, the prevalence of antecedent illnesses, the variability of the host,
and the time over which the causative factors operate. Two distinct
clinical syndromes have been described, viz. kwashiorkor and marasmus.
They occupy the two ends of a spectrum with a mixture of the clinical
features of both in between. The biochemical features also form a
spectrum though they are more evident in kwashiorkor than in
marasmus. It is not unusual to find that a child diagnosed as suffering
from kwashiorkor shows the typical features of marasmus after the
oedema (see 'clinical features') subsides, while a child with nutritional
marasmus often develops oedema and progresses to marasmic
kwashiorkor.

Of the two classical syndromes, kwashiorkor has received a great
deal of interest and attention because of the striking clinical features
and extensive changes in the body's chemistry. However, there are now
clear indications that marasmus is on the increase, especially in the
city slums and shanty towns of the developing countries. The rapid
decline in breast feeding has a great deal to do with this. Moreover,
since marasmus usually occurs at a younger age than kwashiorkor, its
long-term effects are more severe. In both forms of malnutrition,
recognition at an early stage is important in order to avoid the serious
after-effects of established malnutrition. Hence there has been great
interest in accurate classification and especially in identifying early
signs.

Mild-to-Moderate Malnutrition

In defining the stages of malnutrition, two processes have to be taken
into account. These are: (i) the period over which malnutrition occurs
so as to decide whether it is acute or chronic, or acute on chronic. Acute
forms chiefly affect body weight rather than height, whereas in the
chronic form both height and weight are affected. (ii) The aetiological
factors. The classical explanation that kwashiorkor is due to protein
deficiency with relatively adequate energy supply while marasmus is due

to the overall deficiency of proteins and calories arose out of the observations that in countries where roots, tubers and plantain (all with 1-2 per cent protein) form the staple foods, kwashiorkor is more common. This view has been challenged as we saw in the previous section, and the role of infection has been emphasised more in the aetiology of malnutrition.

In every locality the identification of the important aetiological factors is necessary for instituting early intervention. When food is adequate, the organism adapts first of all by reducing growth and the clinical signs are those of such adaptation. Thus, weight gain slows down, and so weight for age has been commonly used to assess the degree of mild to moderate malnutrition. Refinements have been added to this measure in the form of regression lines and various indices like weight/height^2 or weight/height$^{1.6}$. One may question the value of these complexities which require mathematical manipulation.

Reduced growth in adapting to lack of food also affects height. Weight can swing up and down, but obviously this is not the case with height. All that happens is that growth in height slows down and the individual will end up stunted. Catch-up growth in both height and weight can occur if the slowing of growth was temporary, as for example after an acute illness. If dietary deficiency is prolonged catch-up does not occur and the deficit in height becomes fixed and permanent. Thus deficits of height indicate long-standing malnutrition.

Besides growth in height and weight, the body-compartments most affected in malnutrition are those of energy reserve — subcutaneous fat and the protein store of skeletal muscle. Measuring these two body compartments can shed extra light on the pathophysiological mechanisms. Thus, in malnutrition muscle is wasted not only because of lack of protein in the diet, but because muscle is used up to supply energy. Deficient muscle with adequate body fat will be one indication of protein deficiency. Conversely, adequate muscle with lack of fat suggests lack of energy reserve and not necessarily calorie deficiency.

The adaptive changes to dietary deficiency are not always successful. For example, we know that undernourished individuals have a predisposition to infectious illnesses. Diarrhoeal disease is not only more prevalent in undernourished children, but also tends to be more severe. In Zaire, childhood infections, especially measles, were traced in more than half the children in the weeks immediately preceding an outbreak of kwashiorkor. Associated deficiencies besides those of protein and calories also occur with malnutrition. Hence in identifying early malnutrition it is useful to remember that the differing proportions of protein and calories in the diet, the duration of malnutrition, the associated deficiency of other nutrients, and the effects of infectious illnesses together give rise to a wide spectrum of signs and symptoms.

The need for simplification. Malnutrition is a complex situation involving the interaction of several factors with varying degrees of severity. Inevitably, this has led to many complex methods of classification. Such methods, however useful as research tools, cannot be easily taught to auxiliaries and village health workers, for whom a more simplified and action-oriented approach is necessary. With this need in mind, several simple methods of measuring nutritional status have been evolved. The Wellcome classification is one such simple method for the diagnosis of clinical malnutrition.

Wellcome Classification

Weight	Oedema	
(% of standard)	Present	Absent
80–60	Kwashiorkor	Undernourished
< 60	Marasmic kwashiorkor	Marasmus

For children within the community who are at risk of mild-moderate malnutrition a similar simple tool for the selection of early cases is required. The Gomez classification was first suggested in the late 'fifties as a method of diagnosing mild-moderate forms of malnutrition in the community and for the early identification of marasmus. The classification is based on weights of healthy American children under the age of five years, and the fiftieth percentile is taken as the standard. Malnutrition is graded into three degrees of increasing severity according to the percentage reduction in weight from the standard.

Gomez Classification

First degree malnutrition	—	< 80% of the standard
Second " "	—	< 70% " " "
Third " "	—	< 60% " " "

The Gomez classification has been criticised on two counts. Firstly, it does not take height into consideration. Secondly, in some communities more than half the children fall in the category of third degree malnutrition, and health workers doubted whether the growth standards of one community were applicable to another. With further experience it is now realised that the place on the growth chart where a child's weight falls is not so important as the shape of his growth curve compared to the standard. This knowledge has helped to remove a great deal of controversy and contributed to the spread of weight charts in most countries of the Third World. When Morley described the first weight chart in Nigeria it carried two curves. The upper curve represented mean weights of children from the upper social class and the lower curve did the same for the lower social class. Since then there has been considerable debate with regard to local standards, definition of 'normal' children and so on. This controversy delayed the development of local weight charts. When it was realised that it was the shape of the child's weight curve as compared to normal which was important and not the actual weight, the use of weight charts based on the Boston standards received a great boost. More recently a working party convened by the World Health Organisation has developed a weight chart for international use. In this chart (Figure 1.11), the upper line represents the fiftieth percentile of the weights of English boys and the lower line the third percentile of the weights of French girls. Thus, further development in the concept first proposed by Gomez and colleagues has facilitated the regular use of weight charts in children's clinics in many countries.

Present experience shows that it is possible to train auxiliaries and even lesser-trained health personnel in the charting and interpretation of growth records. In the present state of development of health services even these are not available in all areas and the new trend is to train part-time village health workers, the candidates for which are not always literate. A yet simpler way of assessing nutritional status of children is therefore required. Circumference of the mid-arm as an indicator of muscle mass has been used as one of the parameters for measuring nutritional status. It is known that in the normal child between the ages of one and five years the arm circumference changes very little. Here then is a parameter which is age independent. The first practical use of this concept was made during the Biafran war for selecting malnourished individuals in the refugee camps for intensive rehabilitation. The arm circumference was compared with the height of the individual and grades of malnutrition were identified in accordance with the percentage reduction in the arm circumference. More recently, Shakir has shown in Baghdad children that measurement of the arm circumference was a useful tool for diagnosing malnutrition. Children whose arm circumference was less than 75 per cent of the standard also had a body weight less than 60 per cent of the Harvard standard in nine cases out of ten. The practical value of this observation is that primary school children and illiterate village health workers can be trained to use a string or a strip of plastic with a mark and colours in green (over 14.0 cm), yellow (12.5 to 14.0 cm) and red (less than 12.5 cm) for assessing malnutrition in village children (Figure 1.13).

Figure 1.13: Part-time Village Health Worker Using the Arm Band Method to Identify Beneficiaries of a Village Feeding Programme

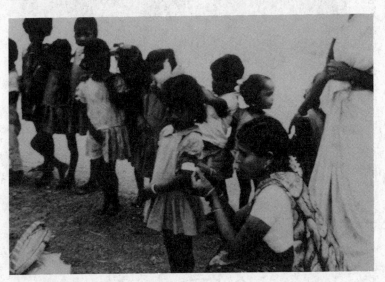

Clinical Features

In the early stage of malnutrition clinical signs are few and even absent, and diagnosis requires both biochemical tests as well as anthropometric measurements.

In the severe forms growth failure is obvious. In addition, activity is reduced so that the child is listless and apathetic or irritable. Because of this irritability communication between the child and the parents is minimal, and often resentment builds up. There is also discolouration of hair and skin, anaemia of varying severity, signs of associated deficiencies and presence of infection.

Figure 1.14a: Characteristic Features of Kwashiorkor

Figure 1.14b: Child with Kwashiorkor*

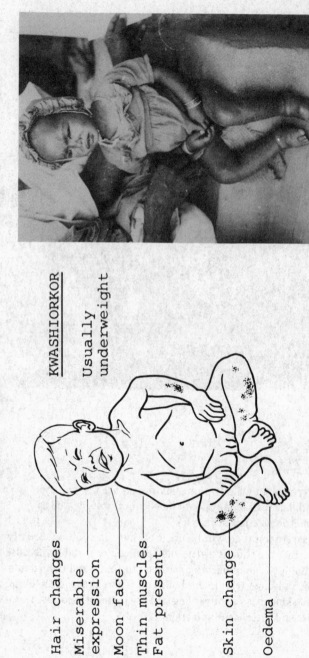

*Note the miserable expression, the skin lesions on the left leg and the swollen, oedematous ankles.

KWASHIORKOR

Usually underweight

Hair changes

Miserable expression

Moon face

Thin muscles
Fat present

Skin change

Oedema

Kwashiorkor

Kwashiorkor (Figure 1.14) presents with failure to thrive, oedema, apathy, anorexia, diarrhoea and discolouration of the skin and hair.

The general appearance may be that of typical 'sugar baby', with chubby features and bloated body, so that at the time parents may think it is doing well and cannot be convinced that the child is malnourished.

Failure in growth is marked and weight is reduced in spite of the presence of oedema. Varying degrees of muscle wasting are present. The discolouration of hair and skin give the child a characteristic 'red baby' appearance. In addition various forms of skin disorder can also occur.

Oedema is the characteristic clinical sign of kwashiorkor. It appears first on the dorsum of the feet and ankles and spreads upwards to involve the rest of the body. Oedema fluid can represent 5-20 per cent of body weight so that change in the appearance of the child when the fluid is lost can be striking.

Another major characteristic is the change in personality. Most children with kwashiorkor are apathetic or extremely irritable and miserable. Marked improvement occurs on treatment, and many clinicians stress that the return of the smile is the first sign of improvement.

Physiological functions of the various systems are markedly disturbed, with diarrhoea, electrolyte disturbance, circulatory insufficiency, metabolic imbalance and poor renal function. Hence the child with kwashiorkor should be thought of as an emergency in need of intensive medical and nursing care and not just simply malnourished.

Marasmus (Figure 1.15)

This usually occurs in younger children, with failure to thrive. Affected children are under height, as well as weight, for their age. In appearance they are shrunken and wizened due to lack of subcutaneous fat. Until recently kwashiorkor had aroused maximum interest and attention, but it is now increasingly realised that marasmus is the fast growing disease of the large urban slums and shanty towns attached to the cities of the Third World. The sharp increase in bottle feeding amongst the urban poor and the new migrants to the cities is largely responsible for the increase in the incidence of marasmus. Since the slums and shanty towns are also the 'septic fringes' of the cities, the marasmic child commonly suffers from infections of all sorts, though more commonly respiratory and diarrhoeal illnesses.

Figure 1.15a: Typical Features of Marasmus

Figure 1.15b: Child with Marasmus

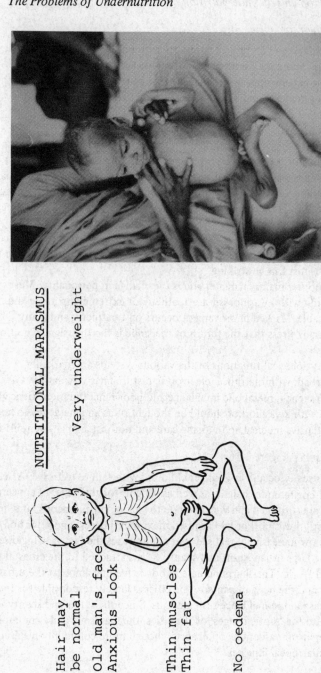

NUTRITIONAL MARASMUS

Very underweight

Hair may
be normal

Old man's face
Anxious look

Thin muscles
Thin fat

No oedema

Associated Deficiencies

Nutritional deficiency is very rarely restricted to just one or two nutrients. As a rule the deficiency is generalised so that, besides clinical signs of protein and calorie deficiency, there also exist signs of vitamin and other deficiencies.

Many of the illnesses which precipitate protein-calorie malnutrition also provoke loss of nutrients from the body in the same way as they cause a negative nitrogen balance. The type of local food staple, the age of the child and the time over which the child's diet has been insufficient also help to determine the severity and the nature of associated deficiencies, the most common of which are those of the fat-soluble and water-soluble vitamins and of iron.

Xerophthalmia

In the rice-eating countries of South East Asia, deficiency of vitamin A is endemic and is commonly associated with protein-energy malnutrition. In Indonesia about three-quarters of all cases of kwashiorkor also have the eye disease, xerophthalmia. In Thailand, the incidence is forty per cent, but in East and West Africa and in the West Indies the reported incidence is only about one per cent. Clinical deficiency is only the tip of the iceberg, because in endemic areas children with PEM but no clinical eye signs invariably have low levels of vitamin A and depleted liver stores of the vitamin. Presence of eye lesions therefore indicates a long-standing deficiency and is often a danger signal, since the mortality from PEM in such cases is about four times that of children who have no ocular lesions.

Rickets

Rickets is a common finding in cases of PEM from the urban slums and inner city areas. It is more common in the younger child suffering from marasmus than in the older child suffering from kwashiorkor. Rickets, like xerophthalmia, has been more commonly reported from S.E. Asia, where prevalence rates of 15-18 per cent have been recorded. It is a rare finding in East and West Africa and in the West Indies.

Vitamin B Deficiency

Laboratory tests show that children with PEM have depleted stores of the water-soluble vitamins, chiefly those of the B group. In many cases, there are visible manifestations of deficiency disease. The effects of protein deficiency on the mucosal lining of the mouth, skin and gastro-intestinal tract may alter the classic manifestations of B-complex deficiency. Many vitamins act as co-enzymes in several key metabolic reactions in the cell. Their deficiency, together with the deficiency of protein and calories, can seriously disrupt cell function. Supplementation with vitamins during treatment is essential in order to replenish tissue stores and to ensure optimal function of the new tissue generated during growth.

Anaemia

Anaemia is also a common accompaniment of protein-calorie malnutrition. The commonest form of anaemia is of the iron deficiency type, which is as expected, since iron deficiency is so widespread in the tropics. But there is very little response to iron therapy until such time as recovery from malnutrition also begins. In several countries the anaemia is reported to respond better to folic acid and B_{12} than to iron. Hence during treatment it is important to administer several haematinics, the more so because treatment is usually based on an artificial formula containing high energy and protein, and not on a complete food as such.

Pathological Features and Changes in Metabolism

As the fat stores of the body are consumed and muscle tissue depleted total body water increases as a percentage of body weight. A direct relationship can be demonstrated between weight deficit and total body water. A proportionate increase occurs in the extracellular fluid. On recovery, some of the excess extracellular fluid is taken up by the regenerating cells and some is lost by diuresis.

As the tissue cells break down, potassium and nitrogen are lost in equal proportions initially. Later on, there is increased loss of potassium in diarrhoeal stools causing a cellular deficit of potassium. The total body protein is severely reduced, ranging from 55 per cent to 80 per cent (average 59 per cent) of normal. Non-collagen protein is depleted more than collagen protein. Muscle mass is greatly diminished and may be only 30 per cent of normal for age. Similarly, in marasmus, body fat may fall as low as 5 per cent of total body weight, compared to the normal of 19 per cent.

Changes in the Digestive System

Liver. A fatty liver is characteristic of kwashiorkor. The fat content of the liver may be as high as 50 per cent of the total wet weight. As recovery occurs, fat gradually disappears. Electron microscopy of liver tissue obtained by biopsy reveals that after three weeks of treatment on a balanced diet, the liver cells are still not visibly normal, even though serum protein levels have reached normal levels. Recognisable liver pathology can be identified even after 10 to 12 weeks of treatment. Total recovery eventually occurs and liver biopsy 5 years later has shown no signs of residual damage, using light microscopy. There are two obvious reasons for the fatty liver. There is an increased flux of fatty acids from adipose tissue for the production of energy. At the same time there is decreased hepatic synthesis of β-lipoproteins which normally transport triglycerides from the liver. The synthesis of the apoprotein part of this fat-transporting mechanism is particularly sensitive to lack of protein in the diet.

Pancreas. There is a marked atrophy of the acinar cells, and exocrine secretion is reduced in keeping with the atrophic changes. Enzyme activity of the pancreatic juice has been reported to be as low as 50 per cent of normal. Recovery takes place within the first few days of instituting treatment. Investigation of B cell function reveals that in both kwashiorkor and marasmus insulin secretion is abnormally low after oral administration of glucose. Improvement occurs after 3 to 6 weeks of treatment, though there are instances where an abnormal response persisted up to 10 months after recovery from malnutrition.

Gastro-intestinal tract. Striking morphological changes occur in the jejunum, especially in kwashiorkor. In particular, villous atrophy may be severe. Enzyme activity is reduced within the cells in keeping with the morphological changes. The enzymes most affected are the ones located in the brush border. Of these lactase has been studied extensively because it is more severely affected and because most diets used for recovery are based on milk and contain large quantities of lactose. Besides these morphological changes, the small intestine also suffers from bacterial overgrowth with invasion of the proximal gut by the bacterial flora of the distal part of the small intestine.

The changes in gut morphology, together with reduction in the amounts of pancreatic enzymes and bacterial overgrowth of the small gut, are together responsible for the common occurrence of diarrhoea in malnutrition. Impairment of absorption is also likely, but, in most cases, is not severe enough to interfere with recovery. For example, up to 33 g of fat containing unsaturated fatty acids is tolerated daily by malnourished children. Clinical experience with diets containing large quantities of vegetable fat supports this observation and cottonseed oil is now a common ingredient of many dietary regimens. With regard to protein digestion, it has been found that even though faecal nitrogen excretion in malnourished children is on average twice the normal, there is no serious malabsorption of nitrogen. More than three-quarters of the nitrogen in the diet is absorbed and is usually sufficient to allow the initiation of a cure except in very severe diarrhoea. Intolerance of lactose can present a serious problem at times, but even here the incidence of practical difficulties with feeding is small (less than 10 per cent). Thus, knowledge of the alteration in digestion and absorption is helpful in dealing with complications when they arise, but these are rare and in most cases it is possible to treat and rehabilitate children suffering from malnutrition without the need for sophisticated laboratory support.

Heart. The heart muscle suffers in the general atrophy of all muscle tissue. Cardiac output is reduced in accord with the reduced body metabolism. Institution of treatment, by stimulating metabolism, can often precipitate congestive cardiac failure. The salt content of the therapeutic diet and presence of anaemia may contribute in causing congestive cardiac failure.

Haemopoietic system. A mild to moderate anaemia is a common accompaniment of PEM. Deficiency of nutrients like protein, iron and folic acid, in addition to bone marrow depression due to infection, are all undoubtedly involved in the aetiology of the anaemia. Parasitic infections like malaria and hookworm are also of relative importance in the tropics where childhood malnutrition is common. The fall in haemoglobin is related to reduction in the erythrocyte mass which commences with tissue wasting and loss of body weight. Megaloblastic changes in the bone marrow frequently occur and in some areas, e.g. the Sudan, the anaemia is reported to respond to folic acid administration. In the first few days of treatment, with regeneration of plasma proteins and the expansion of plasma volume, the concentration of haemoglobin may fall further, accentuating the anaemia.

Muscle. The muscle compartment of the body comprises a large mass of protein which is both labile as well as sensitive to dietary changes. Muscle wasting is an early result of PEM. At recovery the average muscle mass is usually about twice that during the malnourished state.

Muscle and fat biopsies in malnourished Peruvian infants at the time of admission and again 4 to 9 months later, after recovery, show that there is a gross reduction of muscle cell size in malnourished infants. Improvement takes place with recovery, but the cell size continues to remain subnormal after recovery. Thus clinical recovery does not always reflect cellular maturity.

Metabolic Changes

Carbohydrate metabolism. Low blood sugar is a common accompaniment of PEM. Two types of hypoglycaemia have been identified — asymptomatic, from which recovery occurs with feeding, and the profound irreversible type, associated with severe malnutrition, hypothermia or infection. As a general rule, if the child has hypothermia it is almost certain that hypoglycaemia is also present.

Fat metabolism. Fat malabsorption is common in PEM, but the degree is rarely serious enough to cause steatorrhoea (fatty diarrhoea). Probably the most serious result of fat malabsorption is the impairment of absorption of fat-soluble vitamins. It has been found that vegetable fats are better absorbed than animal fats and this is the rationale behind the use of cottonseed oil as a source of energy in the treatment of kwashiorkor.

Protein metabolism. Protein digestion, though inefficient because of low levels of pancreatic trypsin, is sufficient for recovery to occur when an adequate diet is being fed. On average, absorption of nitrogen from a milk-based diet is 70 to 80 per cent as compared to 90 per cent in the normal child. Similarly, in the absence of complicating infection, nitrogen is well retained, being in the range of 20 to 40 per cent of the intake. Thus, protein repletion through a greatly enhanced anabolism is usual as soon as sufficient protein is given. Nitrogen retention continues to be high until a normal growth rate has been attained.

Albumin synthesis and its level in plasma are very sensitive to protein intake. There is an immediate fall when dietary deficiency occurs, and a rise when the deficiency is corrected. Serum albumin levels are also sensitive to infection. The longitudinal study of Ugandan children showed that a combination of respiratory infection, diarrhoea and malaria caused a dramatic fall in serum albumin.

Defence Mechanisms

The child with malnutrition is very susceptible to infection. The body's defences are unable to mount an adequate response to microbial challenge so that the mildest infection tends to spread and become life-threatening. In severe cases the clinical response to infection, like fever and phagocytosis, may be absent and the first sign of widespread infection may be sudden deterioration in the general condition, refusal to take food and hypothermia.

Studies of the body's defence mechanisms reveal adequate capacity for humoral immunity. Thus immunoglobulin levels in the blood are normal and there are normal numbers and proportions of B lymphocytes, which produce immunoglobulins. Secretory IgA in salivary and nasopharyngeal secretions, and the gastrointestinal tract, is reduced and does not rise in response to antigenic challenge. In contrast, cellular immunity (T cell function) is profoundly impaired. T-lymphocytes are reduced in number to about a third of normal and various tests of their functions also show impairment. In keeping with the lowered cellular immunity, all lymphoid organs show atrophy, especially the thymus. Phagocytic function is also inefficient and several workers have emphasised its correlation with iron deficiency, especially lower levels of serum transferrin. The mechanisms of interaction between nutrition and infection are further discussed in Chapter 3.

Management

The objectives of treatment are:

(i)   To achieve rapid regeneration of tissues and institute cure of the malnutrition.
(ii) To treat complications and reduce case fatality. The present mortality rates are as high as 20 to 40 per cent.
(iii) To achieve rehabilitation on a well-balanced solid diet.
(iv) To prevent relapse and future deterioration through education of the parents.
(v)   To achieve long-term follow-up with a view to helping the child and his family.

The principle of treatment is to raise the nutritional level of the child by administering adequate calories, proteins, minerals and vitamins and to get him to eat a well-balanced diet prepared from local foods in as short a time as possible.

During recovery a linear relationship can be demonstrated between velocity of weight gain and the intake of energy, varying from virtually no weight gain at 100 kcal/kg/day to a maximum at 200 kcal/kg/day. It is necessary that the diet should provide at least 150 kcal/kg/day to initiate recovery. In the past a great deal of emphasis was put on the amount of protein in the diet. It has now been realised that 2 g/kg body weight of protein is required for the regeneration of tissues, and amounts in excess of 3 g/kg/day are wasted and burnt as energy. Thus provision of adequate calories is more important than large amounts of protein. Carbohydrates in the form of sugar or starch will be bulky and the best way of providing energy is in the form of fat, especially vegetable oil, which is better absorbed.

During convalescence, when appetite has returned, a child eating a balanced diet consumes 160 kcals/kg and 2 to 3 g protein/kg daily. The early days, however, are critical, as the child is desperately ill, the body's metabolic processes are at an ebb and additionally there may be complications like hypothermia, hypoglycaemia and infection. Moreover, anorexia and irritability make the feeding difficult. A liquid diet fed through a nasogastric tube is helpful at this stage and most clinicians find a milk-based formula, with the addition of casein and oil to increase the protein and calorie content, useful for initiating treatment. Originally, dried skimmed milk powder was used as the basis of the formula. It was fortified with casein, cottonseed oil and sucrose to provide the required protein and calories. Full cream dried powdered milk has also been used in the same way. The various ingredients are mixed in proportions shown in Table 1.14.

Table 1.14: High Energy — High Protein Formulae for Initiating the Treatment of PEM

	Casein skim milk diet	Casein full cream milk diet
Casein (g)	35	30
Dried skimmed milk (g)	35	—
Full cream milk (g)	—	60
Sugar (g)	35	30
Edible oil (g)	70	45
Water (ml)	1000	1000

Potassium 1.0 g and magnesium 0.5 g are added to each 100 ml of the above diet to replenish tissue stores and to provide the requirements of the regenerating cells. The formula is administered at the rate of 110 ml/kg/day. Supplements of vitamin and iron are also necessary to make up the deficits and to provide the daily requirements.

As recovery occurs oedema is gradually lost — in a week or so — and appetite returns. At this stage solids can be introduced gradually until the child is able to take ordinary food.

Several complications arise. Of these the most important are hypothermia, hypoglycaemia and sepsis. Persistent hypothermia even with frequent feeding is a danger signal and is often due to underlying infection. Severe diarrhoea due to lactose intolerance occurs in a small number of cases and responds well to the removal of lactose from the child's diet. After a week or so on a lactose-free diet ordinary milk feeds can be tolerated, though in some cases lactose intolerance is known to persist for several weeks.

Hospital Management

The trend hitherto has been to consider PEM as any acute disease and to treat it in hospital. More recently doubts have been raised with regard to the suitability of the hospital for treating all forms of malnutrition. The cost of hospital treatment is high. In countries where childhood malnutrition is common it is not unusual to find 20 to 40 per cent of hospital beds taken up by people with malnutrition. Cross infection is hospital is usual and often a child recovers from malnutrition only to succumb to some infection. Hence case fatality for hospital treatment is high. Moreover, after all this investment in time, effort and cost, children are usually discharged to that same home environment where the disorder first started.

However, a case can be made for treating severe cases *initially* in hospital. These children are desperately ill; many of them are likely to develop complications and are in need of intensive care.

Home Management

There is now a growing experience of the benefits of treating the child with mild to moderate malnutrition at home, within the family environment and the community. In several imaginative programmes successful use has been made of the health visitor and village health worker to achieve rehabilitation of such cases at home using locally available foods. The parents see their children improve with better feeding and come to appreciate the importance of many of the locally available foods in the weaning of children. Moreover, the food is prepared utilising only the resources of the village home. Under supervision, the mother learns skills which will benefit other children in the family as well as the neighbourhood. This change of emphasis from the hospital ward to the home and family environment for the management of malnutrition has, in turn, led to several innovative approaches for dealing with the problem at the community level.

Innovative Approaches

Nutrition Rehabilitation Centres (Figure 1.16a, b and c)

The nutrition rehabilitation centre was first described in the sixties as a convalescent place or staging post between the hospital ward and the home. Two advantages were immediately obvious. Firstly, they took the pressure off the crowded hospital wards where treatment costs were becoming prohibitive. Secondly, nutrition education of the mothers was easier to organise and more effective in the relatively quiet environment of the nutrition rehabilitation centre in comparison with the rush in the acute paediatric ward. Soon the activities of the nutrition rehabilitation centre were expanded to include training in mothercraft, in improved techniques of farming, raising poultry, environmental sanitation and other similar activities. When the activities of the nutrition rehabilitation centre were integrated with those of the out-patient services and under-fives clinics, they became the focal points of maternal and child health work and of disseminating new knowledge in the community. Mothers admitted to such centres often later take on the role of advisers in child feeding in their immediate neighbourhood.

The nutrition rehabilitation centre is basically a school for parents who come together as either residents or day visitors to learn about better ways of feeding their children. They learn by participation and by observing their children thrive on foods which they have cooked at the centre. The facilities consist of a residential unit or a ward with a kitchen and a plot of land where the foods used in the daily cooking are grown. The emphasis is on cooking multi-mixes which provide adequate calories and protein in manageable bulk.

A recent evaluation in Uganda, Peru, Haiti and Guatemala has proved that children attending these centres *do* show improved growth and nutrition recuperation in an impressive way. The cost per child per day ranged from US $372 in Haiti to US $876 in Guatemala and was ten to forty times less than that of hospitalisation. However, the effect of the nutrition rehabilitation centre on the knowledge of the mother was not always impressive.

Community-Centred Approaches

Several shortcomings of the nutrition rehabilitation centre are obvious, even though it is a significant advance compared to the hospital ward for the treatment of malnutrition. Only a small proportion of all children suffering from malnutrition in the community are brought to a health facility for treatment, and only a proportion of these will be

Figure 1.16: Nutrition Rehabilitation Centres

a: The communal kitchen

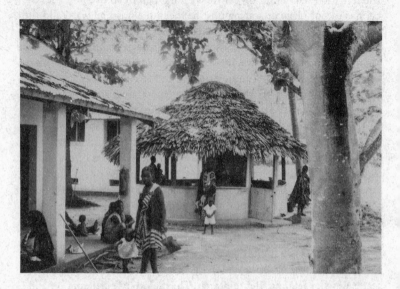

b: The residential area

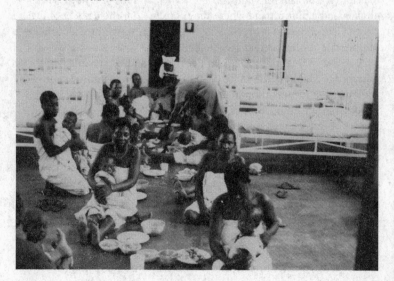

c: Group discussion (with vegetable garden in the background)

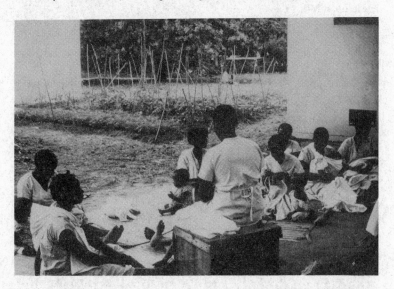

eventually admitted to the nutrition rehabilitation centre. Thus a centre can provide only limited coverage. It is physically impossible to provide one centre for each village in a country. Secondly, nutrition rehabilitation centres treat children after malnutrition has occurred. What most countries need is a preventive/promotive activity.

Due to these reasons, health workers have experimented with more community-centred approaches. For this purpose a new look at the problem of childhood malnutrition and our methods of dealing with it is necessary. Traditionally we tend to think of malnutrition as any other disease in which the problem is at the family level and the management is also aimed at the level of the family. But malnutrition is a problem at the level of the community and is the consequence of the prevailing state of cultural, social and technical development. A community which is able to feed its children is in a healthier state of development than one which cannot. One must therefore search for solutions within the community on the principle that 'the state of

Figure 1.17: Members of a Village Women's Organisation Producing Hyderabad Mix

a: Roasting wheat, Bengal grain and groundnuts

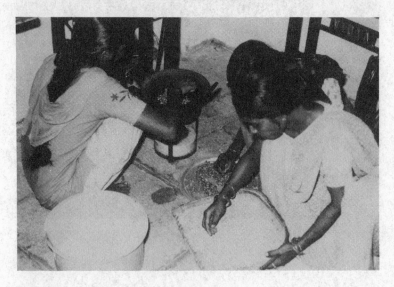

b: Grinding the roasted grain into flour

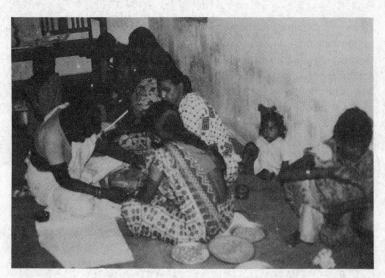

Figure 1.18: Volunteer Labour in a Community Programme for Improving Agricultural Production. Damming a Brook in Jamkhed

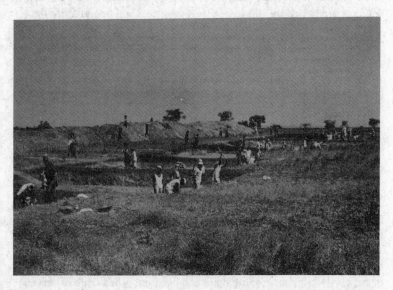

nutrition is determined by what people do and not by what they get'. Amongst the community-based programmes are those for increasing productivity at the village level, preparation of weaning diets from local foods in the form of multi-mixes, child feeding programmes out of community effort, identification of beneficiaries for community assistance by village health workers using simple techniques, and other similar activities. Many of these activities supplement the effects of services like the under-fives clinics described earlier, and together prepare the community for programmes of integrated development. Thus, in Hyderabad (India) the village community has mobilised itself to create farmers' groups who raise crops on communal plots; the women in turn process these foods into a nourishing multi-mix, the village health workers identify children in need of food supplementation and all these activities are strongly supported by a network of community health activities. In Jamkhed (India) the community increases its agricultural potential by building earth dams across streams, and young farmers' clubs raise crops for a village feeding programme which is supervised by village health committees and operated by the village health workers.

These are some of the new approaches. But they are all in experimental stages and operating within defined boundaries. For them to spread both nationally and internationally requires a new breed of professional capable of identifying the social, ecological and other root causes of nutritional disorders, and of working with the community to find solutions.

Vitamins in Health and Disease

Vitamin A and Xerophthalmia

Xerophthalmia and its most serious manifestation, keratomalacia, have probably occurred in badly fed communities throughout human history. The condition was well-known to Hippocrates who described the use of liver in its treatment. Throughout the nineteenth century a number of papers describing xerophthalmia had been published from different parts of the world, including during the Irish potato famine in 1848. An important observation was made during the first world war in Denmark which helped to associate deficiency of vitamin A with xerophthalmia. Butter was replaced by margarine in the Danish diet during the war years and defatted milk was commonly used for infant feeding, with the result that there was an outbreak of xerophthalmia and keratomalacia amongst Danish children.

The size of the problem on a global scale was not fully appreciated until 1962 when a survey sponsored by WHO showed vitamin A deficiency to be a major cause of blindness in children in all the 30 countries in South East Asia, Africa and Latin America included in this survey. It is estimated that every year 85,000 cases of blindness occur in children due to xerophthalmia, chiefly in the rice-eating countries of South East Asia. In India, several nutrition surveys suggest that 8 to 10 per cent of rural children between six months and six years have signs of vitamin A deficiency, and of the country's estimated blind population of 4.5 million, about a quarter or a third owe their disability to the after-effects of vitamin A deficiency. A nutrition survey in Jordan showed blood levels of vitamin A within the 'deficit' range ($< 10 \mu g/100$ ml) in 5 per cent and 'low' ($10 \mu g$–$20 \mu g/100$ ml) in a further 39 per cent of the children examined. Thus,

clinical vitamin A deficiency represents only the tip of the iceberg.
There are many more amongst the apparently healthy community with
poor body stores who can be precipitated into an acute deficiency
state.

Many children with clinical vitamin A deficiency have advanced eye
lesions when first seen. This may be due to the rapid progress of lesions
once they are established, or because of difficulties in access to medical
facilities. In Central Java, out of 8,000 cases of xerophthalmia seen in
1960 in an eye clinic, 8 per cent had advanced lesions likely to cause
loss of vision and twice this number had moderate lesions which were
expected to respond to treatment, but leaving residual corneal scarring.
Furthermore, not all those blinded by xerophthalmia survive.
Deficiency of vitamin A is commonly associated with protein-calorie
malnutrition and other nutritional deficiencies. The common
observation is that for every survivor from advanced xerophthalmia
there is another who dies.

Epidemiology

The peak prevalence of xerophthalmia is in the third and fourth years
of life. In this respect it differs from PEM, which has its highest
frequency at the age of 18 months. It is a condition seen almost always
in a growing child. Depletion of body stores takes much longer in
adults, since growth has ceased and utilisation of vitamin A for the
growth of new cells is much less.

In the search for a specific dietary cause of xerophthalmia it is often
forgotten that vitamin A deficiency is a social disease affecting the
poorest sections of the community who are forced to live on a
monotonous diet and suffer recurrent illnesses. Socio-economic
development in many countries has resulted in a fall in the incidence
of xerophthalmia and the condition is now rare in Hong Kong,
Singapore and Taiwan, where it used to be common. Social upheavals,
on the other hand, cause widespread hardships and precipitate
xerophthalmia and other deficiency disorders, as happened in
Bangladesh and South Vietnam.

Vitamin A deficiency is especially common in the rice-eating areas
of South East Asia where 2-8 per cent of all preschool children may
show clinical manifestations. The wheat-eating countries of West Asia
and North Africa have fewer cases. In tropical Africa, on the other
hand, xerophthalmia is not at all common and only a few cases are seen,
usually in association with long-standing PEM. In West Africa the
common use of red palm oil in cooking acts as a major protective

measure against vitamin A deficiency.

The primary cause of low body stores of vitamin A is dietary deficiency caused by a monotonous diet made up almost entirely of cereal. Protective foods with high β-carotene content like amaranth, carrots, spinach and paw-paw are not offered because of local traditions and beliefs that such foods give rise to diarrhoea in children or because of ignorance. The result is a low intake of vitamin A or its precursor. Dietary surveys in several rural communities in South East Asia show that the average daily intake of vitamin A in children is 70 μg compared to the requirement of 300 μg. By comparison the average daily intake in affluent western communities is 1,200 to 3,000 μg. Similar dietary surveys in countries of the Near and Far East reveal an average daily intake of 300 to 900 μg, but in some poor communities it is as low as 150 μg.

Some children with such chronic dietary deficiency may progress to show clinical signs of xerophthalmia or Bitot's spots (shiny, grey triangular spots on the conjunctiva) either alone or in combination with protein-calorie malnutrition. More commonly an intercurrent illness leads to a sudden loss of vitamin A from the body followed by acute onset of clinical disease. Several disease processes are known to cause a loss of vitamin A from the body. In tuberculosis, pneumonia, urinary tract infections and other chronic diseases massive excretion of the vitamin in the urine has been recorded. For example, in adult patients suffering from pneumonia such a loss has been estimated to be in the range of 1,000 μg/day. In children, measles, whooping cough and recurrent diarrhoea are common precipitating factors. Epidemics of these illnesses in rural communities leave in their wake many children with acute vitamin A deficiency.

It is not widely known that ocular pathology can progress rapidly. A child brought to an outpatient clinic with Bitot's spots and some corneal involvement can deteriorate within a day and develop keratomalacia and total destruction of the cornea unless vitamin A is administered in adequate doses and immediate steps are taken to protect the eye and to correct coexisting nutritional deficiencies.

Seasonal variations in prevalence rates have been reported from many countries. These variations are not always explained by changes in intake. Possibly they are related to seasonal variations in growth or in the seasonal incidence of intercurrent illnesses. In most countries where xerophthalmia is endemic there is a summer peak in incidence rates following diarrhoeal illnesses and a winter peak coinciding with respiratory infections.

Physiology of Vitamin A

Vitamin A is obtained in the diet either as preformed vitamin A or as β-carotene. In the average western diet half of the vitamin A activity is provided as carotene and the other half as preformed vitamin A. In the peasant communities of the developing world β-carotene is the major source of the vitamin. The cells of the intestinal mucosa convert β-carotene to vitamin A. Two molecules of β-carotene give rise to one of retinol, though the theoretical yield is hardly ever reached and, in general, the activity of β-carotene is about a sixth of vitamin A.

Preformed vitamin A occurs in food in the form of long chain retinyl esters. These are hydrolysed in the intestinal lumen by means of pancreatic hydrolase and also by a similar enzyme present on the brush border. Within the mucosal cells the retinol is rapidly re-esterified and later transported in the lymphatics within chylomicrons. When it reaches the vascular compartment, the retinyl esters are removed from the circulation almost entirely by the liver, and stored in the liver parenchymal cells as fat globules. When required, vitamin A is mobilised from the liver cells and carried bound to a specific trans-port protein − the retinol binding protein (RBP). In the circulation, RBP occurs in combination with pre-albumin in the form of a protein-protein complex. In protein deficiency states the release of vitamin A from hepatic stores is affected because of defective hepatic production of carrier proteins including RBP. It is likely that the low levels of vitamin A in PEM reflect a functional impairment in hepatic release of vitamin A rather than vitamin deficiency as such, for the hepatic release of the vitamin is improved with adequate feeding without supplementary vitamin A.

The role of vitamin A in the production of visual purple and for the integrity of the conjunctival and corneal epithelium is well established. Almost all the clinical signs of vitamin A deficiency are related to vision and the eye, viz. night blindness, dryness of conjunctiva, Bitot's spots, keratomalacia with scarring and destruction of the cornea resulting in blindness (Figure 1.19a and b). Recent work in laboratory animals indicates that vitamin A is necessary for growth; in fact measurement of growth has been used as an assay for vitamin A activity in the rat. Abnormalities in RNA metabolism and protein synthesis do occur in severe vitamin A deficiency, but do not cause striking clinical signs as in the case of xerophthalmia.

Approaches to Prevention

Clinical vitamin A deficiency needs urgent treatment because of the

Figure 1.19: Keratomalacia

a: Child with Keratomalacia Causing Blindness in the Left Eye

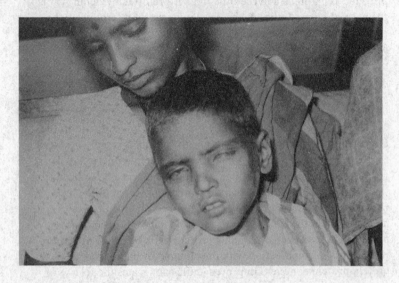

b: Close-up of Keratomalacia — There is a Softening and Destruction of the Cornea

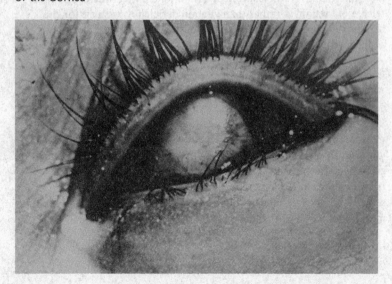

tendency for rapid deterioration in the eye. Vitamin A is necessary especially when there are obvious signs of PEM and if ocular lesions are advanced. Parenteral administration is also necessary if there is associated diarrhoea and vomiting and where oral administration cannot be relied upon. In such cases intramuscular injection of the water-miscible form 30,000 i.u. daily is required for several days. In protein deficient states intramuscular administration of oily vitamin A is not effective and such preparations are best avoided.

There is clearly a need for health and nutrition education in all developing countries, but this is a slow process and urgent solutions are necessary. This is more so because blindness due to xerophthalmia is preventable. Amongst the various approaches developed the nutrition rehabilitation centre and mass prophylaxis with vitamin A are the most promising. The nutrition rehabilitation centre was described in the previous section and is best suited for rehabilitation of children suffering from xerophthalmia complicated by PEM. Parents of children who have been admitted to such a centre become useful sources of knowledge on child feeding in their neighbourhood. Moreover, the centre itself provides opportunities for the training of village health workers and auxiliaries. The first nutrition rehabilitation centre established in 1970 to deal with xerophthalmia in South India has been successful and has become the springboard of a large community programme.

In the last few years an imaginative approach has been tried out in several countries for the prevention of xerophthalmia. This approach is based on the fact that vitamin A is a depot vitamin and it should therefore be possible to fill the depot. After several field trials it has been found that a dose of 200,000 i.u. of vitamin A in oil given orally is tolerated well. When administered every six months such a dose is able to maintain adequate tissue stores and protects against xerophthalmia. Laboratory studies with labelled vitamin A have shown that about 47 per cent of the orally administered dose in oil is retained in the body. Observations in communities with well developed programmes of mass prophylaxis have shown a significant fall in the incidence of ocular manifestations of vitamin A deficiency. Several countries have now adopted this method for the prevention of childhood blindness.

Rickets and Metabolic Bone Disease

Rickets is primarily a disease of children in the first two years of life when rapid skeletal growth causes increased requirements of vitamin D and minerals. It is a disease of calcium and phosphorus metabolism

Figure 1.20: Rickets

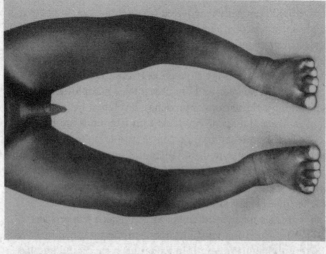

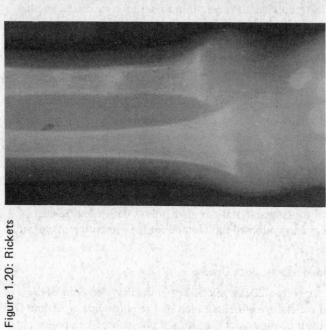

a: X-ray of the wrist showing the abnormalities of the growing ends of the radius and ulna in rickets. The cartilage is fragmented and hollowed out and little calcification is apparent.

b: Bowed legs of a child with infantile rickets.

which occurs when infants and children receive insufficient vitamin D.

The clinical effects of vitamin D deficiency are mainly seen in the growing parts of the bone, the epiphyses of long bones (Figure 1.20 a and b) and the costochondral junctions. In addition the bones of the body become soft due to poor mineralisation and deformities like bow-legs occur on weight-bearing. In the active stage of rickets, the child looks ill. He is pale, irritable, sleepless and at times may suffer from tetany and convulsions. But the disease is very rarely fatal in itself, except that respiratory infections tend to be more frequent in rickets. The most important effects of the disease are retarded physical growth and skeletal deformities due to a disorder of bone calcification.

Epidemiology

Historical. Rickets was known in ancient times and it is most likely that sporadic cases occurred in the larger cities throughout the Middle Ages. The first full description of the disease was written in the seventeenth century by the English physician Glisson. Throughout the eighteenth and first half of the nineteenth century rickets was common in the cities of western and central Europe. It reached its peak prevalence in the latter half of the nineteenth century and in the first decade of the present century. The rise of textile industries in England led to the employment of women and children and crowded living conditions in the cities. As slums grew, sunlight became scarcer in the lives of many of the working population. This, added to the unhygienic methods of child rearing such as swaddling and being kept indoors without opportunity for outdoor play led to a great rise in the incidence of rickets. In industrial cities of Britain the disease was almost universal and came to be known as the 'English disease', even though it was equally common elsewhere. In 1907, in the hospitals of Paris one of every two children between 6 months and 3 years of age showed evidence of rickets. In Boston, it was estimated that 80 per cent of the children of poorer classes suffered from the disease. In 1921 it was estimated that fully three-fourths of the children in large cities like New York showed some evidence of rickets. At about the same time a third of infants born in Glasgow were said to have it.

When the beneficial effects of sunlight and cod liver oil were recognised it became possible to bring rickets under control and the disease has now been virtually eliminated from many of the larger cities of industrial nations. In Britain the principal early measure against rickets was cod liver oil, issued through the infant welfare clinics. Throughout the twenties and the thirties the use of cod liver oil was promoted by the infant welfare services, with the result that at the outbreak of the second world war rickets had become a rare disease in Britain. About this time further nutritional measures were introduced in the form of a free supply of cod liver oil and vitamin D for infants and pregnant mothers, fortification of infant foods with vitamin D, enrichment of margarine with vitamins A and D, and addition of calcium carbonate to wheat flour. As a result of these measures rickets became rare towards the end of the war.

Resurgence of rickets in recent years. In the early sixties rickets reappeared in Britain. This time it was mainly confined to immigrants from the Indian subcontinent and the West Indies. An incidence of 30 per cent overt rickets and osteomalacia in children and adult women has been reported in some studies. If abnormal biochemical findings are also included, the prevalence of vitamin D deficiency rises to 74 per cent in children and 53 per cent in adults. Several studies of the dietary habits of immigrant groups show that there is a prompt abandonment of breast feeding even though in the homeland the baby not breast-fed has little chance of survival. In contrast, the adult feeding habits remain virtually unchanged.

In spite of these different dietary habits, the nutrient content of the diet of the immigrant child, including the intake of vitamin D, was not different from that of a control group of Scottish children. There is also no significant difference in the diets of rachitic and non-rachitic immigrant children. It would therefore seem that the non-dietary source of vitamin D is important. These observations are borne out by studies of vitamin D status in immigrant groups in comparison with that of communities in their countries of origin. Such studies show that, despite the similarity in diets, Asians in Britain have a higher incidence of biochemical abnormalities suggestive of rickets than similar groups in the homeland. Exposure to sunlight is thus an important aetiological factor in vitamin D deficiency. Women and children amongst the immigrant groups are more at risk because of staying indoors and, especially in the latter, the traditional way of dressing which exposes few body parts to sunlight.

Rickets in the Tropics and Subtropics

In many countries of sub-Saharan Africa rickets is rare. As the cities grow and industry develops it is likely that many of these countries will experience a rising incidence of rickets.

In India, a frequency of 0.9 per cent in urban and 1.5 per cent in

rural children of low socio-economic groups has been reported
the sprawling slums of the large cities in Asia and Latin Americ
likely to be the major factors in the incidence of rickets. Osteon
in women, on the other hand, is relatively common. In New Dell
hospital has reported admitting 60 people with advanced osteom.acia
per year. In the majority the presenting signs are those of vague pain in
the back and legs, but in about 10 per cent tetany is the first symptom.
Most are women in the reproductive period and in many of them
repeated pregnancies are contributory factors.

Rickets is relatively more common in the Middle East where women
observe the Muslim tradition of 'purdah' and parents are reluctant to
expose children to the burning sun. In a survey in four countries of
North Africa (Morocco, Algeria, Tunisia, Libya), sponsored by WHO
in 1965, rickets was noted in 10 to 11 per cent of children admitted to
hospital or attending outpatient clinics in Morocco and Algeria. In
Tunisia and Libya the frequency was 3 and 5 per cent respectively in
similar groups of children.

Physiological Mechanisms

Very few natural foods provide vitamin D (Table 1.15), with the
exception of fish. Fish liver oils have traditionally been major sources
of the vitamin, before a synthetic vitamin became widely available.
Fish obtain their vitamin D from eating plankton exposed to sunlight
on the surface of the sea.

Table 1.15: Sources of Vitamin D

(Recommended intake 10 µg (400 i.u.))

Food	Range µg/100 g
Fish	5–45
Egg (whole)	1.25–1.5
Egg (yolk)	4–10
Margarine (vitaminised)	2–9
Butter	0.25–2.5
Cheese	About 0.3
Milk	0.1
Cereals, vegetables and fruit	No vitamin D
Meat and white fish	Insignificant amounts

Many people obtain no vitamin D from the diet and their entire source of the vitamin is from the skin through exposure to sunlight. The average British diet provides 2.89 μg of vitamin D per day compared to the daily requirement of 10 μg. Of this amount in the diet about a third comes from margarine enriched with the vitamin. Fish and eggs together provide another third and the remainder is obtained from milk and milk products. Thus, for the average Briton, exposure to sunlight provides twice as much vitamin as that in the diet. It has been estimated that the cheeks of a European infant (area 20 cm^2) can synthesise daily about 10 μg of vitamin D if adequately exposed — sufficient protection against rickets.

7-dehydrocholesterol is the precursor of vitamin D in the skin. On exposure to the ultraviolet rays in sunlight, it is converted to cholecalciferol (vitamin D$_3$). The exact mechanism by which it is absorbed from the skin is not known. As we have noted, dietary sources are only required when a person is shielded from effective sunlight by clothing, housing conditions or smog.

On absorption from the skin or the gut, vitamin D accumulates rapidly in the liver where it undergoes hydroxylation yielding 25-OD-D$_3$, which is the major circulating metabolite of the vitamin. Further hydroxylation occurs in the kidney giving rise to 1-25-(OH)$_2$-D$_3$ which is the active form of vitamin D and behaves like a calcium and phosphate-mobilising hormone in the body.

Dietary and serum calcium levels play an important role in regulating the production of 1-25-(OH)$_2$-D$_3$ by the kidney. Low intake of calcium, causing low serum levels, stimulates the production of 1-25-(OH)$_2$-D$_3$ whereas diets high in calcium, leading to increased serum calcium concentration, suppress the production of 1-25-(OH)$_2$-D$_3$. Instead, there is a production of another metabolite, 24,25-(OH)$_2$-D$_3$. Thus, at normal serum calcium levels the kidney produces both 1-25-(OH)$_2$-D$_3$ and 24,25-(OH)$_2$-D$_3$. In hypocalcaemia there is preferential production of 1-25-(OH)$_2$-D$_3$ and in hypercalcaemia of 24,25-(OH)$_2$-D$_3$. This effect is mediated through the parathyroid hormone. Low serum calcium levels stimulate parathyroid hormone secretion which, in turn, increases the production of 1-25-(OH)$_2$-D$_3$ by the kidney.

The above observations are borne out by experiments in human volunteers. After the administration of oral vitamin D there is a delay of 16 to 20 hours before increased calcium uptake occurs. The time lag can be reduced to 6 hours by giving 25-OH-D$_3$, but the time lag still occurs indicating that it is 1-25-(OH)$_2$-D$_3$ which is the active compound.

Under its influence calcium is absorbed from the gut and transported across mucosal cells in assocation with calcium-binding protein. The absorbed calcium then reaches the osteoid seams and growing cartilage of bone where it is incorporated.

With intakes below 600 mg per day most individuals are in negative calcium balance. On a dietary intake of 600 to 1,000 mg a normal adult absorbs about half the ingested calcium and the net absorption varies little over this range. When calcium intakes fall below 500 mg adaptive mechanisms increase the proportion which is absorbed. In severe calcium restriction the efficiency of absorption can reach up to 70 to 80 per cent, mediated through increased production of $1\text{-}25\text{-}(OH)_2\text{-}D_3$.

The daily intake of calcium in the diet and its source (Table 1.16) both vary from one population group to another and also from one individual to another depending upon dietary habits.

Table 1.16: Calcium Content of Some Common Foods

Food	Range mg/100 g or 100 ml
Milk — cow's fresh whole	120
Cheese — from whole or skimmed milk	80—1200
Eggs — fresh, whole	50—60
Beef, mutton, pork and poultry	3—24
Pulses — raw dried	40—200
Vegetables — raw green leafy	25—250
Whole wheat — full extraction	30—40
Wheat flour — 70% extraction	13—20
Rice — raw, polished	4—10
Maize	5—18
Millet	20—50
Potatoes — raw	7—10

In a global survey of calcium intake it was found that there were four broad groups of countries.

(i) Most of Europe and North America. The average intake of calcium is 900 mg/head/day. Of this 70—90 per cent is derived from milk and its products.
(ii) Southern Europe and central South America. The average intake

is 650 to 800 mg/head/day. Of this 50–70 per cent is from milk and milk products, but vegetables also make an important contribution.

(iii) Chile, India, South Africa, Turkey, Egypt. The average intake is 350 to 500 mg/head/day. Of this, milk supplies 30–65 per cent, but cereals, pulses, vegetables and nuts also make a contribution.

(iv)   Japan. Intake is 350 mg or less derived fairly evenly from cereals, pulses, nuts, vegetables.

Osteomalacia

This is characteristically found in women who live on cereal diets lacking in calcium and, for one reason or another, are mainly confined indoors. When they go out they are covered with clothing which prevents adequate exposure to sunlight. The most striking accounts have come from Northern India and the Middle East where the condition is encountered in its more severe forms. More recently cases have been described from immigrant Asian women in Britain. Symptoms consist of body pains which are often misdiagnosed as psychosomatic. In advanced cases characteristic bone deformities occur and skeletal X-rays show demineralisation of bone.

Osteomalacia is also likely to occur in the elderly. The efficiency of calcium absorption tends to decrease with age, so higher intakes, as much as 900 mg/day, may be necessary for the elderly to remain in calcium balance. Because of ignorance, lack of resources, physical disability with eating, and relative immobilisation they are deficient both in calcium and vitamin D. An incidence of 8 per cent has been reported in 200 elderly women consecutively admitted to hospital in Glasgow. Further observations are needed on the frequency of osteomalacia in the elderly in both temperate and warm countries.

Hypercalcaemia

Excess intake of vitamin D can lead to hypercalcaemia, especially in susceptible infants. The widespread tendency to enrich infant foods with vitamin D increases the risk, especially when we know that large inaccuracies do occur in the measurement of milk powder. In the fifties several cases of infantile hypercalcaemia were diagnosed in Western Europe and North America. This led to a recommendation for considerable reduction in the vitamin D content of infant foods. However, the risk is still present, especially with the availability of highly potent and concentrated forms of vitamin D on the market and the tendency for parents to ask for 'tonics'.

Clinical Manifestation of Rickets

Bony changes and skeletal deformities are the most striking characteristics of rickets, even though other clinical features like irritability, excessive sweating, refusal to eat and a tendency for bronchopneumonia have been found to be commonly present in the rachitic child. There is extension and widening of the epiphyses, more easily noticed at the lower end of the radius (Figure 1.22) and at the costo-chondral junctions of ribs. If the disease occurs before the age of six months there is also softening of skull bones. Circumscribed areas in the membranous bones of the skull remain unossified, yielding to pressure with the fingers and giving a characteristic feel, similar to that of pressing on parchment.

Late signs are bony deformities in lower extremities, like bow-legs or knock-knees, and a transverse depression of the chest which deepens on expiration. All these deformities can be explained by the softening of bones which bend under stress, either that of weight-bearing or by muscle traction. Frontal bossing of the skull, late closure of the anterior fontanelle and various bony deformities are other stigmata of rickets.

Treatment and Prevention

Life threatening situations like hypocalcaemic tetany need to be treated with intramuscular administration of a large dose of vitamin D (15,000 μg) in oil. Most cases of rickets respond well to oral administration of 250 μg of vitamin D daily for a period of 4-6 weeks. Radiological improvement is seen in 2 to 3 weeks, though biochemical tests continue to remain abnormal for a long time.

As past experience shows rickets is preventable. The problem is now mainly confined to a section of the community with large families living in slums and inner city areas. Mothers in such families do not use infant welfare services and are unresponsive to health visitors. Amongst immigrant families there are added difficulties because of language and cultural differences. Moreover, exposure to sunlight in dull and cold climates and in crowded cities is not always possible. A multiple approach through education, provision of fortified foods and periodic administration of vitamin D through home visits, as in the case of xerophthalmia, is most likely to succeed in such circumstances.

Deficiencies of Vitamins of the B Group

The vitamins of the B group act as co-factors or activators of enzymes and thus have a key role in metabolism. Enzymes involved in metabolic activity vary a great deal in their functions. Some require only their main proteins to be active, others require the presence of co-factors. In some cases these co-factors are simple metallic ions and in others they are more complex molecules. In the latter case they are termed co-enzymes, and the vitamins of the B group are mainly co-enzymes or precursors of such co-enzymes.

Most co-enzymes bind loosely to the protein portion of the apoenzyme, but some like thiamine bind more firmly. Some co-enzymes serve as receptors for the products of enzyme reaction. For example, folic acid serves as a receptor of methyl groups and one carbon fragment in the synthesis of purine and in the metabolism of several amino acids. Some co-enzymes act as electron or proton receptors. Thus, riboflavin acts as a receptor of hydrogen atoms in the oxidation-reduction reactions within the mitochondria for the liberation of energy. Some co-enzymes, on the other hand, act as structural supports to the enzyme molecule, exposing the active sites or changing their configuration for optimal chemical reaction without directly participating in reactions.

Deficiencies of vitamins in the B group arise for various reasons. The commonest cause is dietary, caused by either inadequate consumption of food or by eating processed foods in which the vitamin concerned may have been removed or destroyed. Rarer causes are poor intestinal absorption or a deficiency of transport protein needed for the transfer of the vitamin across the gut mucosa. At the cellular level, the co-factors may not be transported across the cell membrane, transport within the cell may be defective, or it may not be converted to the form needed to activate apoenzymes. The co-factor may not bind adequately to the apoenzyme because of a defect in the protein binding site or because some other compound is competing. Deficiencies at the cellular level give rise to abnormal metabolism with the formation of toxic by-products.

Physiological Roles of Niacin (nicotinamide; nicotinic acid)

The vitamins of the B group are widely distributed in nature. In addition, many of them are synthesised by intestinal bacteria, so that in a healthy individual eating a mixed diet deficiencies are rare. In spite of this, widespread deficiencies reaching epidemic proportions have occurred not very long ago with regard to several vitamins. These are pellagra due to niacin deficiency and beri-beri due to lack of thiamine in the diet. In addition, megaloblastic anaemia of pregnancy caused by deficiency of folic acid is still common in many parts of the developing world today. Both pellagra and beri-beri, which once affected tens of thousands of people, are now on the decline, but the causative factors and the circumstances in which they occur still continue to exist and the potential for future outbreaks remains.

Niacin (nicotinamide) is widely distributed in plant and animal foods (Table 1.17).

Table 1.17: Sources of Niacin

(Recommended daily intake 6.6 mg/1000 kcal)	
Food	Range (mg/100 g of edible portion)
Wheat bran (mainly outer bran)	25.0—46
Wheat flour (70% extraction)	1.0
Wheat flour (British 1956 regulation)	1.5
Rice (lightly milled)	2.0—4.5
Rice (highly milled)	1.0—1.6
Sorghum	2.5—3.5
Pulses	1.5—3.0
Millets	1.3—3.2
Maize*	0.2—1.5
Sorghum*	2.5—3.5
Groundnuts	16.0
Green leafy vegetables	0.2—1.5

* Staple foods commonly associated with pellagra

In the tissues tryptophan can be converted to niacin and the presence of animal protein in the diet helps to protect against deficiency of niacin. Milk, meat and eggs protect against pellagra because of their tryptophan content. It has been estimated that 60 mg of tryptophan can give rise to 1 mg of niacin. Presumably such a conversion only occurs when tryptophan is in excess and there is a need for niacin. Increasing amounts of tryptophan are first used to achieve nitrogen balance, next to restore blood pyridine nucleotide and then for conversion into niacin. It is customary to take into account both the niacin content of food as well as the amount of tryptophan present in order to determine the 'niacin equivalents' of diets. The amount of niacin required is related to the total calories consumed and the recommended daily intake is 6.6 niacin equivalents for every 1000 kcal consumed per day. In the normal European diet about half the niacin comes from proteins of animal origin.

In some foods, like maize and possibly the potato, niacin occurs in a bound form and cannot be absorbed in the gut. It can be liberated from the bound form by treatment with alkali. In Mexico and in the diets of many American Indian communities maize is first treated with lime water before being used as food. This helps to liberate niacin from the bound form and increases the amount of utilisable niacin in maize, which explains the low incidence of niacin deficiency in these communities.

Cooking does not destroy niacin except that considerable amounts may be dissolved in the water used for cooking and in the fluids which come out of meats during cooking. If these fluids are discarded instead of being consumed, considerable amounts of niacin may be lost.

Niacin has an essential role in the oxidative mechanisms by which the chemical energy present in the molecules of carbohydrate, fat and protein is liberated and made available for cellular metabolism. It is the precursor of two co-enzymes, NAD (nicotinamide adenine dinucleotide) and NADP (nicotinamide adenine dinucleotide phosphate) which act as hydrogen acceptors in oxidation-reduction reactions. The energy thus released is trapped by the synthesis of high-energy phosphate bonds, and the two co-enzymes participate in these reactions as well.

Pellagra

This is a deficiency disorder caused by lack of niacin. It occurs in poor peasant communities which subsist mainly on maize with very little variety in the diet. The typical clinical features are loss of weight, debility, an erythematous rash characteristically affecting the parts of the body exposed to sunlight, gastrointestinal disturbances and mental changes. Diarrhoea and mental change are not always present, especially in early cases, and often the mental symptoms consist of depression or confusion.

The disease first made its appearance in Europe after the introduction of maize from the New World; with maize it spread through Europe from Spain to France, Italy, Central Europe, Rumania and Turkey. It later spread into Egypt and tropical Africa. In the first decade of the present century, pellagra was a major disease in the United States, chiefly affecting the poor whites and negro farm labourers in the South. In 1928, 6,969 deaths were recorded from pellagra in the US and by 1930 20,000 cases were reported in the state of Georgia alone. Because of its sudden and widespread occurrence it was then thought to be a new epidemic disease of infective origin. Many observers have ascribed the sudden appearance of pellagra in the US to the wide-scale poverty and depression following upon the Civil War and the development of large milling concerns which marketed finely ground corn flour, which looked and tasted better, but lacked the germ and its vitamins. The commercial milling of maize in the US made a poor diet even poorer and was the major precipitating factor in the occurrence of pellagra.

Elsewhere similar disasters were recorded. In Rumania, in 1932, 55,013 cases were recorded with 1,654 deaths. In some villages where maize was the staple food providing something like 75 per cent of total calories, up to 10 per cent of the population suffered from pellagra every spring. In Lesotho in 1956 it was reported as the most common deficiency disease. During the warm months 15 per cent of the population were affected. In South Africa, in the Bantu reserve areas, about half the patients attending the outpatient clinics have pellagra skin lesions, and more than half of all Bantu patients admitted to mental hospitals are suffering from pellagra in one form or another.

In 1927, the nature of pellagra as a deficiency disorder was established, and the use of milk as a protective food was well known. Liver extract for the treatment of pellagra was available in 1937, and it was not long before niacin was synthesised and widely available. At the same time the governments of many countries instituted preventive programmes. In the US, agricultural extension programmes promoted the development of small farms instead of concentrating on the growing of cotton. In France, government action discouraged the cultivation of maize. In Italy, government subsidies established bakeries to sell bread made from wheat. Similarly, in Egypt maize was gradually replaced by subsidised wheat and farmers were encouraged to mix maize with wheat or millet.

As a result of these measures, pellagra is now on the decline. It is disappearing from the US and countries of southern Europe and the incidence has decreased in the Middle East, even though it continues to remain endemic in small pockets. Africa is now the only continent where pellagra is still a public health problem. It occurs seasonally in a mild form, the dermatitis recurring each year with the growing season. Recurrent and prolonged niacin deficiency in these communities is a cause of chronic diarrhoea and debility. Intercurrent infections in affected individuals are often fatal. After suffering prolonged niacin deficiency and its various complications many ultimately suffer from dementia.

Recently, pellagra has been reported from rural communities in central South India, where maize is not eaten, but sorghum forms the staple diet. Sorghum is high in leucine and the consumption of large amounts of the staple causes an amino-acid imbalance with secondary lack of tryptophan and niacin deficiency as a consequence. Sorghum fed as 65 per cent of the diet to dogs has been shown to give rise to black tongue, which is the canine equivalent of human pellagra.

Present trends. Pellagra persists in some vulnerable groups like pregnant women and the elderly in peasant societies subsisting on maize. But the disease is nowhere as widespread as the epidemics which affected the United States and southern Europe in the early part of this century. Pellagra is also found in chronic alcoholics and in patients suffering from malabsorption. Tubercular patients who are on poor diets and on long-term treatment with the anti-tubercle drug, isoniazid, may sometimes show clinical signs of deficiency. More recently, pellagrous skin lesions have been reported in the rare Hartnup disease, in which there exists a defect in the transport of tryptophan across mucosal cells resulting in malabsorption and renal loss of this amino acid.

Clinical features of pellagra. The characteristic features of pellagra, in the skin, the digestive and the nervous system, are commonly super-imposed on the general features of undernutrition. Underweight and general debility are often prominent.

The changes in the skin are characteristic and appear symmetrically over those parts of the body which are exposed to the sun. The hands, forearms, face and skin are covered by an erythematous rash resembling sun burn. The lesions burn and itch, and may progress to formation of vesicles which exude fluid causing encrustation and ulceration. Secondary infection often occurs. In long-standing and chronic cases the skin is thick and roughened, with scaling and dark pigmentation.

Diarrhoea is a common but not constant feature. In the advanced case the mouth is sore with a raw tongue and inflamed fissures at the angles of the mouth. The anal canal and rectum may be similarly involved, indicating pathological changes involving the mucous membrane of the lower gastrointestinal tract, causing the intractable diarrhoea. Anxiety and depression are usually present. In the more severe and acute forms delirium is common and the more chronic and long-standing cases also show signs of dementia. Sensory disturbances are common amongst the latter, with consequent loss of position sense and ataxia.

Treatment and prevention. There is prompt response to nicotinamide 100 mg given 4-hourly by mouth, with general improvement in mental condition and disappearance of diarrhoea and the skin rash. Because of the strong likelihood of other associated deficiencies, other vitamins of the B group and a well-balanced diet are also necessary. In those acute cases with delirium and excitement, both nicotinamide and the other vitamins need to be given by injection, together with nasogastric feeding.

The disappearance of pellagra from the southern US and many of the countries of Europe demonstrates the effectiveness of preventive measures, and the better understanding of nutritional requirements. In peasant societies, fortification of maize flour with nicotinic acid on a national scale may not be effective because most food is processed in the home. It has been shown that 120 g of groundnuts a day will protect an adult against pellagra. Better extension services and nutrition education in rural societies aimed at the consumption of a mixed diet in addition to national fortification programmes will help to eradicate this eminently preventable deficiency disorder.

Thiamine

All animal and plant tissues contain thiamine, but the more important sources are cereals, peas, beans and other pulses, and yeast. Green vegetables, fruits, dairy products and meat contain appreciable amounts of thiamine, but they are not rich sources (Table 1.18).

In the cereals, thiamine is chiefly present in the outer layers of the grain which get removed as bran during milling for the making of white flour or rice. Moreover, in the case of rice, the removal of outer layers of the grain makes the remaining thiamine more accessible for dissolution in water. Since the common practice is to wash rice prior to cooking, a large part of the remaining thiamine in milled rice is therefore lost during washing. On the other hand, if rice is parboiled, as is the custom in rural communities of South India, the vitamin is driven into the inner layers of the grain and the losses during milling are minimised.

Thiamine is stable at high temperatures. Losses in cooking occur only when the water used for cooking is discarded, since it contains a large proportion of this highly soluble vitamin. Thiamine is denatured if baking powder is used or if soda is added in the cooking of vegetables.

Table 1.18: Sources of Thiamine

(Recommended daily intake 0.4 mg/1000 kcal)

Food	Range (mg/100 g of edible portion)
Whole wheat	0.4
Pulses	0.4
Millets	0.4
Rice (home pounded)	0.08—1.4
Rice (parboiled and milled)	0.11
Bran (rice or wheat)	2—4
Milk, cow's	0.04
Eggs	0.10—0.15
Meat	0.16—0.30
Poor sources associated with deficiency	
White bread (70% extraction)	0.05—0.07
Rice (milled)	0.02—0.04

Several foods contain anti-thiamine factors which can alter the biological activity of the vitamin. The viscera of fresh water fish and shell fish as well as several micro-organisms contain substances which catalyse the decomposition of thiamine. These substances are thermo-labile and are destroyed during cooking, thereby preserving the vitamin. On the other hand various vegetables and plants also contain anti-thiamine factors which are thermostable and do not get destroyed on cooking.

In many rural Thai communities where thiamine deficiency is endemic studies of nutritional status and food intake have shown that not only is the diet deficient in thiamine, but that the raw fermented fish, which is consumed in large quantities, and the habit of chewing fermented tea leaves as stimulants also make the deficiency worse because of their anti-thiamine activity.

In the healthy individual, thiamine is well absorbed by the intestinal mucosa. At high concentration, absorption is by passive diffusion; at low concentration by active transport. In chronic alcoholics absorption of thiamine is defective, due to associated folate deficiency and malnutrition. Correction of malnutrition and supplementation with folic acid greatly improve thiamine absorption in these individuals.

At the cellular level, thiamine plays an important role in energy metabolism. It participates as a co-enzyme in the metabolism of α-keto acids, like pyruvate and the keto analogues of leucine, isoleucine and valine. It also participates in several important metabolic processes like the pentose phosphate shunt, yielding NADPH. Besides these metabolic roles, thiamine has a specific role in neurophysiology independent of its co-enzyme function.

Beri-beri is a nutritional disorder caused by deficiency of thiamine. The classical descriptions mention two types – wet and dry beri-beri – according to the body systems which are principally involved. The wet type is so called because oedema and symptoms of congestive cardiac failure predominate. In the dry form the prominent signs are those of involvement of the nervous system. The common mode of presentation, however, is the subacute type in which the characteristics of both wet and dry beri-beri are present. A serious form occurs in young breast-fed infants whose mothers are themselves deficient in thiamine. This *infantile form* is at present the commonest variety encountered. It occurs in infants less than 6 months old who are acutely ill with dyspnoea, cold extremities, weak pulse and aphonia. X-rays show an enlarged heart shadow. There is a dramatic response to injection of thiamine.

Beri-beri has been described in various communities in South East Asia where rice is the staple diet. In fact, what maize is to pellagra, rice is to beri-beri, especially the highly milled variety in which thiamine-containing outer layers of the grain have been removed as bran. The disease has also been described in fishing communities on the coast of Newfoundland and Labrador living on a diet principally composed of white wheat flour, salted meat and molasses during the long winter months from October to April.

Early descriptions of beri-beri can be found in medical literature in 1645 and 1835. It was in the last quarter of the nineteenth century that beri-beri appeared suddenly in many countries of South East Asia. It continued as a formidable problem both in extent and severity for about half a century and is now present only in isolated pockets in several South East Asian countries. It would seem that the causative factors in the sudden appearance of beri-beri were the introduction of steam driven rice mills, so that the use of white, highly milled rice became popular. About the same time several estates and mines employing a large labour force adopted the practice of issuing rice rations as part of the wages for the labourers. Similar practice was also common in the armed forces and barracks. In the affected families, rice was often eaten alone or with little else. For example it has been noted that rice provided between 2,500 to 3,000 kcalories daily, indicating the large quantities in which it was consumed.

Several observations finally led to the understanding of beri-beri as being a deficiency disease. Epidemiological studies in Malaysia showed that there were three sharply defined communities in the country. The Malays were predominantly agricultural and rural. They grew their own rice and consumed it after home pounding; beri-beri was rare amongst them. The Tamils used parboiled rice, as is the custom in South India. Again beri-beri was rare in this group. The Chinese, on the other hand, were mainly migrant labourers, who consumed white rice provided by their employer. This group was highly prone to beri-beri, with heavy mortality. Further research in the laboratory revealed the protective effect of rice bran. Later thiamine was identified and synthesised. Improved understanding of the nutritional requirements, the wide-scale availability of synthetic thiamine, and fortification of rice by mixing it with the grain coated with thiamine have all helped to reduce the incidence of beri-beri. Socio-economic development has also resulted in an improved quality of dietary intake and is another factor in the decline of beri-beri.

Riboflavin is widely distributed in nature, dairy produce and foods of animal origin being comparatively richer sources than cereals and plant foods (Table 1.17). It is heat stable and is not destroyed by cooking, apart from the losses which can occur if the water used for cooking is discarded.

Riboflavin is the precursor of the various flavo-proteins which act as co-enzymes in many oxidation-reduction reactions.

Clinical and biochemical evidence of widespread deficiency is lacking. However, signs of riboflavin deficiency occur in conjunction with other nutritional disorders and should be looked for when other deficiencies occur.

Clinically, riboflavin deficiency causes angular stomatitis, broken skin and mucous surfaces around the mouth which may become infected with the fungus candida albicans and develop whitish crusts. The tongue is raw. Eating and swallowing are painful and food intake is further reduced because of it. All the above respond to oral administration of riboflavin 20 mg daily.

Table 1.19: Sources of Riboflavin

(Recommended daily intake 0.55 mg/1000 kcal)	
Food	Range (mg/100 g of edible portion)
Wheat bran	0.5
Wheat and barley, whole grain	0.12—0.25
Maize, whole grain	0.1
Millets	0.1 —0.15
Pulses	0.1 —0.3
Fish	0.2 —0.4
Meat	0.1 —0.3
Eggs	0.3 —0.5
Milk, fresh cow's	0.15
Green leafy vegetables	0.05—0.30
Maize meal*	0.02—0.1
Rice, milled*	0.03—0.05
Wheat flour, 70% extraction*	0.03—0.05

*Poor sources

Pyridoxine

This is widely distributed in nature, with meat, liver, vegetables and the outer coats of cereals being rich sources of the vitamin. It participates as a co-factor in a large number of enzymes concerned with amino acid metabolism, though it is now suggested that the main function of pyridoxine is to stabilise the structure of enzymes rather than act as a co-factor. The metabolic usefulness of pyridoxine can be appreciated by the fact the pyridoxine carrying enzymes are involved, in one way or another, in the synthesis and catabolism of all amino acids.

A primary deficiency due to inadequate nutrition is rare, but should be suspected in the presence of other nutritional disorders. In laboratory animals pyridoxine deficiency is characterised by a large number of abnormalities of amino acid metabolism. Poor growth, anaemia, convulsions, decreased antibody formation and renal, hepatic and skin lesions have been described.

Deficiencies can occur through restricted diets, as happened some years ago in infants who were fed a brand of baby food in which pyridoxine had been destroyed through heating. An outbreak of convulsions amongst these infants showed that pyridoxine is an essential nutrient for the developing nervous system. Since then it has been shown that there is a familial tendency in some individuals for higher than normal requirements of pyridoxine. During infancy, they required supplementation with pyridoxine to protect against the risk of seizures, which cannot be controlled by the usual anticonvulsants. Some cases of chronic anaemia not responsive to the usual haematinics respond to pyridoxine, indicating that the vitamin overcomes some unknown defect in haemoglobin synthesis. In susceptible women, oral contraceptives are known to induce changes in tryptophan metabolism which are corrected by administration of pyridoxine. Such metabolic disturbances are common in undernourished communities and supplements of pyridoxine may have to be considered in these circumstances. In more recent years it has been shown that many of the neurological side effects of drugs like isoniazid, cycloserine, hydrallazine and penicillamine can be prevented by pyridoxine. These drugs form complexes with pyridoxine making it unavailable to the tissues.

Summary

This account of vitamin deficiencies serves as a reminder of the dangers of a monotonous diet, especially when the staple has been processed in a way which removes important nutrients. The individual grain of cereal is not only a source of calories, but also contains sufficient vitamins to metabolise the calories present. When this equilibrium is disturbed by technology, as for example removal of the bran, or by bad cooking methods, like discarding the fluids in which the food has been cooked, deficiencies arise. The advent of technology, resulting in the consumption of processed foods, may disturb the balance in nature by selective denaturation of one or more nutrients. There is also the added risk of altering feeding habits through promotion and through the so-called convenience foods. In the interaction between man and nature for obtaining nutrients, food technology, if not correctly applied, can give rise to widespread deficiencies as has happened in the past with pellagra and beri-beri, and more recently with infant feeding.

Nutritional Anaemias

Nutritional anaemias comprise the second most common group of deficiency disorders after protein-calorie malnutrition. Nutritional anaemia is defined as anaemia which occurs when there is a deficiency of one or more of the essential nutrients required for the synthesis of

haemoglobin and the production of erythrocytes. Several nutrients are
required for erythropoiesis.

Iron, folic acid, vitamin B_{12}, protein, pyridoxine, vitamin C, copper
and possibly vitamin E are all necessary for the proper function of the
bone marrow. Iron is an essential component of haemoglobin and a
large proportion of nutritional anaemia in the world is caused by its
deficiency. Iron deficiency tends to be most common when the intake
is not enough to meet the demands of growth, e.g. in pregnancy, during
infancy and at adolescence. Infections and parasitic infestations are
also important; they may interfere with the activity of the marrow, or
increase erythropoiesis by causing blood loss or haemolysis.

Anaemia due to deficiency of folic acid and vitamin B_{12} is much
less common. Both folic acid and B_{12} play a key role in cellular
metabolism and are needed for the normal development of the
erythrocytes in the bone marrow. Folic acid deficiency is more common
than that of vitamin B_{12}, and is mostly seen during pregnancy, when
the demands of the fetus are added to those of the mother. Apart from
pregnancy, deficiencies of folic acid and B_{12} are rare except in malabsorption and in certain diseases of the bowel.

Prevalence

Anaemia is a common cause of hospital admissions in infants and
young children in most of the developing world. In some countries of
tropical Africa, up to 4 per cent of paediatric admissions are for
anaemia, a figure equivalent to that for admissions due to protein-
calorie malnutrition and investigation; the mortality from anaemia can
be as high as 9 to 10 per cent. The frequency of anaemia in out-patients
is even higher. Of 5,000 patients attending the teaching hospital in
Dar-es-Salaam, the mean haemoglobin value amongst 2,539 men was
8.85 g/100 ml. Among 2,108 women it was 7.86 g/100 ml and in 853
children in the age group 1 to 5 years, it was 6.78 g/100 ml. In
Mauritius, anaemia is the second most important cause of admissions
to hospital and in Sierra Leone up to 40 per cent of adult females
suffer from it.

Community studies have been few and scattered. In one detailed
study spread over seven countries of South America it was found that
iron deficiency occurred in 48 per cent of pregnant women as
compared with 21 per cent non-pregnant women and in 3 per cent of
the males of the same age groups. Anaemia, defined as haemoglobin
less than 11 g/100 ml, was found in 38.5 per cent of pregnant women,
17.3 per cent of non-pregnant women and 3.9 per cent of men. The

prevalence of folic acid and vitamin B_{12} deficiency was much lower and these deficiencies seemed to occur only during pregnancy.

In Gambia, in one longitudinal study, 473 rural children under the age of 5 were examined at intervals of 3 months for a period of 26 months. In that community the common practice is to breast feed all children exclusively for 4 to 6 months, after which cereal pap is introduced and gradually supplemented with sauces of fish, ground nuts or green leaves and boiled rice. The mean haemoglobin value under the age of 1 month was found to be 15.4 g/100 ml. It fell as the children grew older reaching 9.0 g/100 ml at the age of 15 to 24 months, after which there was a slow improvement. These values are lower than those of London children in the worst years of the depression in the thirties and of poor Aberdeen children quoted below. A well-marked seasonal cycle was observed in Gambia. There was a sharp decline in haemoglobin values in the latter part of the wet season, indicating that malaria is a key aetiological factor in this age group. In another study of anaemia in rural women in Gambia a high frequency of iron deficiency was observed. In this group there was a strong association between anaemia and three independent variables — pregnancy, heavy menstrual periods and splenomegaly.

A cross-sectional study of haemoglobin values in 726 children under the age of 5 in several coastal villages in Tanzania showed that anaemia was as common as in Gambia. The mean haemoglobin was 8.3 g/100 ml in the first six months of life, increasing slowly to reach a mean of 9.2 g/100 ml between the ages of 5 and 6 years. Again malaria appeared to be implicated. For example, in the city of Dar-es-Salaam, where malaria transmission is considerably less, the mean haemoglobin values were higher — 10 g/100 ml in the age group 5 to 6 years.

Forty infants under the age of six months with severe anaemia were studied in Dar-es-Salaam. Apart from six who suffered from sickle cell anaemia, all had iron deficiency with little or no iron stores in the bone marrow. A large majority were born to mothers who had received no antenatal care during pregnancy. It was thought that many of these infants were born with poor iron stores and could not cope with the requirements of growth. Episodes of malaria made the existing deficiency worse and precipitated acute anaemia.

Such cross-sectional data are available for many communities, indicating the extensive prevalence of anaemia. Even though there are no symptoms from the anaemia it does contribute to ill-health and reduces productivity. In malarious areas, control measures result in better average levels of haemoglobin. This was the experience in Tanzania after instituting control measures. Also community surveys in India, where malaria eradication programmes have been in operation since the sixties, show higher haemoglobin levels than in countries where malaria is holo-endemic. A cross-sectional study in 544 rural Punjabi children showed a mean haemoglobin level of 11.0 g/100 ml under the age of six months, falling to 9.2 g/100 ml at age 18 to 24 months and rising again to 10.5 g/100 ml at 3 years.

In many affluent societies of Western Europe nutritional anaemia used to be a major public health problem until quite recently. In 1935, a survey of 3,500 individuals from the poorer classes in Aberdeen showed that between the ages of 5 and 23 months the frequency of anaemia was 41 per cent and in 7 per cent the haemoglobin level was less than 10.2 g/100 ml. Between the ages of 2 and 5 years, 32 per cent had haemoglobin levels below 11 g/100 ml. After this age slow improvement occurred until adolescence when, amongst 246 pubertal girls, 1 per cent had haemoglobin levels below 9.6 g/100 ml. Anaemia was not a problem among adult men; women tended to have lower haemoglobin values, especially during pregnancy when 17.5 per cent showed values of less than 9.6 g/100 ml. Thus, three age periods were identified as being at risk, infancy, adolescence, especially in girls, and pregnancy. Since then there has been a marked improvement. Recently a mean haemoglobin value of 11.0 g/100 ml has been recorded in Bristol children between the ages of 3 to 24 months and in Cardiff children a mean value of 12.0 g/100 ml in the second year rising to 12.4 g/100 ml at 5 years has been reported.

The general improvement in diet and in health standards have largely contributed to the falling incidence of anaemia in British children. A similar improvement has also been found in pregnant women since 1940, though early prophylaxis with iron and folic acid has also been responsible for the fall in the incidence of anaemia of pregnancy.

Aetiological Factors

Iron Deficiency

Iron plays an important role in the physiology of the body because of its unique ability to give up or accept electrons and oxygen. This enables a rapid change from the ferrous to the ferric state (reduced to oxidised form) with no expenditure of energy. It has thus a central role in respiration both in the take-up of oxygen in the lungs and also in its utilisation at the cellular level.

A large number of foods contain iron (Table 1.20). The concentration varies in accordance with soil conditions so that a range occurs in most vegetable foods.

Table 1.20: Iron Content of Common Foods

(Recommended intake 10 mg/day)	
Food	Range (mg/100 g)
Liver, raw	6.0–14.0
Beef, mutton, raw	2.0– 4.3
Fish (raw)	0.5– 1.0
Eggs (whole, fresh)	2.0– 3.0
Pulses	1.9–14.0
Millets (raw)	4.0– 5.4
Cereals	9.0 mg
Wheat flour (high extraction)	3.0– 7.0
Wheat flour (low extraction)	0.7– 1.5
Green vegetables	0.4–18.0
Potatoes and root vegetables	0.3– 2.0
Milk	0.1– 0.4

All food iron is present in two main forms:

(i)   Inorganic or non-haem iron, which occurs as ferric hydroxide complexes loosely bound with proteins, amino acids or organic acids. Prior to absorption, this form of iron must be split from its combination with organic molecules and reduced to the ferrous state. This happens during acid-pepsin digestion in the stomach. Reducing substances like vitamin C help in absorption. On the other hand presence of phytates can result in the formation of insoluble salts and prevent absorption. For this reason cereals are a poor source, in spite of their rich iron content. Egg yolk also suffers from a similar disadvantage because of its phosphate content.

(ii) Haem iron, which is bound to porphyrin in haemoglobin and myo-globin. Its absorption is not affected by phytate or phosphate or ascorbic acid. Haem iron is absorbed intact into the intestinal epithelial cells and the iron is split off from the haem moiety within the epithelial cell.

Several ingenious studies with radio-active iron biologically incorporated into foods have helped our understanding of the absorptive mechanisms and the availability of iron from various foods. Thus, iron is better absorbed from veal and fish as compared to wheat. The least absorption is from beans, spinach and maize. In general, a diet providing 10-12 mg of iron per day and in which at least 40 per cent of the iron comes from meat will provide adequate amounts for normal adults. The average diet in the UK in 1976 provided 12 mg of iron daily. Of this 15 per cent was obtained from white bread and another 23 per cent came from pastries and cereal products. Meat provided about a quarter of the total iron intake, so that more than half the iron intake came from bread, wheat flour and meat. In the average diet haem iron contributes only 1 to 3 mg of iron per day and in the poorer peasant communities even less. Non-haem iron which forms the bulk of the dietary iron is far less available.

Absorption of iron takes place mostly in the upper jejunum, though some absorption occurs in all parts of the small intestine and even in the colon. All ferric iron in the food must be first converted to the ferrous form before it can be absorbed. This process commences in the stomach and continues in the small intestine. In people with achlorhydria (inability to produce gastric acid) and patients after gastrectomy operations iron absorption is decreased. Achlorhydria decreases iron absorption by 50 per cent. Such individuals cannot increase absorption when they are iron deficient and must be given supplemental iron.

Iron taken up by the brush border of the internal epithelial cells rapidly passes into mucosal cells. There are two pathways of absorption. Some of the absorbed iron is rapidly conveyed to the serosal surface where it enters the plasma for distribution in the body. Some absorbed iron is deposited in the mucosal cells as ferritin. Formerly it was believed that iron absorption was determined by the amount of ferritin deposited in the mucosal cell. Now it seems more likely that ferritin formation is a consequence of failure to absorb iron. Ferritin deposits are then lost with the mucosal cells when they are exfoliated.

The quantity of iron absorbed in the gut is regulated by two factors, iron stores in the body and the state of activity of the bone marrow. In adults with iron deficiency, 20 per cent of labelled iron can be absorbed compared to less than 10 per cent in controls. In the average Western diet providing between 10-15 mg of iron per day, only 5 to 10 per cent is absorbed. Absorption decreases with advancing age especially after

60 when iron deficiency is common.

Iron absorbed into the blood stream is carried by transferrin which is a specific plasma protein of the β-globulin group. In the adult, the transport system deals with 20 mg of iron daily, which is partly liberated from degraded erythrocytes and partly absorbed iron. The daily turnover of plasma iron is about 35 mg; only a small portion of it is derived from the diet even when absorption has been at a maximum. The total amount of tissue iron in the adult is 300 mg and a significant amount is replaced daily to make good the losses in desquamated cells.

Iron is stored in the body in the form of ferritin and haemosiderin. Both forms are available to replace lost iron, but ferritin is more readily available than haemosiderin. Body stores of iron are distributed as approximately a third in the liver, a third in the marrow and another third between spleen, muscle and other tissues.

The total amount of iron in the body is between 3 and 5 g, almost two-thirds of it in circulating red cells and 3 to 5 per cent as myoglobin and in iron-containing enzymes. In all these forms it occurs as haem iron. The remaining 30 per cent is present as non-haem iron, bound to protein for the purpose of storage and transport.

During pregnancy the placenta is a site of significant iron transfer, especially in the later stages. No significant amount of transferrin crosses the placenta so presumably iron is removed from transferrin and taken up by placental receptors, from whence it is then transferred to the fetus. The iron requirements of pregnancy are approximately 2.4 mg/day over the whole nine months and the total cost of pregnancy is 700 mg. Because of the requirements of pregnancy and losses in menstrual blood, the iron requirements of a woman in the reproductive period of life are at least twice those of a man or of a post-menopausal woman.

At birth, the normal full-sized infant has a high concentration of iron in the liver, almost 10 times that at 1 to 3 years of age. The total iron content of such an infant is 250 mg of which 150 mg is present in the red cell mass, 50 mg in tissues and 50 mg as storage iron. Delayed clamping of the cord after birth can increase the blood volume of the newborn by as much as 100 ml, most of which would be broken down and augment the body stores of iron. In communities where iron deficiency is common, maternal anaemia and poor body stores can lead to a low haemoglobin concentration in the cord blood, poor fetal stores of iron and even anaemia in early infancy. For example, at the maternity hospital in Dar-es-Salaam, 100 consecutive cord blood samples showed a mean haemoglobin value of 9.5 g/100 ml (range 6.2 to 13.8 g/100 ml). The mean of the mothers was 6.8 g/100 ml (range 2.6 to 10.0 g/100 ml). Clearly, many of these infants cannot be expected to have normal tissue stores of iron and are likely to suffer from anaemia in infancy.

In the first two years of life, there is rapid growth, so that birth weight doubles by the age of six months, trebles by the age of 1 year and quadruples by the age of two. There is a parallel increase in blood volume and muscle mass and the demand for iron is high in this age group. The requirement during the first year of life is for 200 mg decreasing to 100 mg in the third year. It continues at that level until the ninth year when the requirement increases concomitant with the growth spurt of puberty. Thus, the body needs of iron are high at two periods of life, infancy and pregnancy. In both, the requirements are about six times those of the adult male.

Folic Acid and Vitamin B_{12}

Both these vitamins are necessary in purine metabolism and for the synthesis of DNA. Deficiency causes a characteristic change in nuclear morphology and tissues with the highest rate of cell multiplication are affected first. Deficiency is accentuated by any condition causing increased rate of cell multiplication. Thus it is commonly associated with pregnancy, infancy, lactation and adolescence. For the same reason, haemolysis and certain parasitic infections make marginal deficiency more acute by increasing the requirements.

The commonest form in which deficiency presents itself is megaloblastic anaemia. Severe megaloblastic anaemia is infrequent in affluent societies and occurs usually as a complication of a co-existing main disease. No accurate figures are available of the prevalence of megaloblastic anaemia in the tropics, and it is possible that the frequency and importance of megaloblastic anaemia have been under-estimated. Deficiency can go undiagnosed because it occurs without anaemia or is masked by another haematological or medical disorder.

Megaloblastic anaemia due to deficiency of folic acid is most common in pregnancy. In developed countries, the incidence of megaloblastic anaemia in pregnant women attending antenatal clinics is between 2.5 and 5 per cent. The incidence of megaloblastic change in the bone marrow and of low serum folate levels is 8 to 10 times higher. The information is very scanty with regard to developing countries and present evidence suggests that the incidence of megaloblastic anaemia in pregnancy may be between 20 and 50 per cent.

In children megaloblastic anaemia is rare in well-nourished communities, except as part of the malabsorption syndrome. In developing countries, megaloblastic anaemia is known to occur in protein-calorie malnutrition, especially in pastoral communities living on goat's milk, which is low in folic acid. With cow's milk, boiling or pasteurisation can result in the loss of 75 per cent of the folate.

Folate deficiency is a commoner cause of megaloblastic anaemia than deficiency of B_{12}, because body stores of folate are more easily depleted than those of B_{12} and even a minor degree of dietary lack or malabsorption can precipitate deficiency. Alcohol and several drugs, including anti-malarials, can interfere with folic acid metabolism and cause a deficiency.

Vitamin B_{12} exists in nature only as a product of synthesis by micro-organisms. Fruit, vegetables, cereals and cereal products are devoid of B_{12} and the usual dietary sources are meat and meat products and, to a lesser extent, milk. Because of its predominantly animal source strict vegetarians invariably develop B_{12} deficiency over a period of many years, unless they take special measures to avoid it.

Many of the naturally occurring folates are labile and easily destroyed by cooking. In the average British diet 16 to 24 per cent of free folate is derived from cow's milk. Liver is a rich source so that even one meal of liver can make a significant contribution to the week's intake. In the past it was thought that only free folate was available to the body, but present evidence suggests that both free and bound forms are available. Approximately half the folate present in food is retained and the remainder excreted regardless of whether it is ingested as mono- or polyglutamate.

The average diet in the UK provides approximately 5 μg/day of vitamin B_{12}. Little is known about average intakes in developing countries and one estimate puts it as between 0.5 to 2.0 μg. The maximum amount of the vitamin that can be absorbed at any given meal is between 1.5 and 3.5 μg. The intake from three well-balanced meals in one day will thus provide enough vitamin B_{12} to meet the daily requirement of 2-5 μg. Even the grossly inadequate diet consumed by some old people contains enough vitamin B_{12} to prevent anaemia and therefore a nutritional cause for a deficiency is rare.

Studies of erythropoiesis in megaloblastic anaemia indicate that ineffective erythropoiesis may represent as much as 63 per cent of total erythroid activity. The bone marrow is capable of sustaining erythropoiesis at up to seven times the normal rate, but the proliferative effort only results in an increased number of abnormal cells, which may be destroyed within the marrow or, if delivered into the circulation, are short-lived. The net result is that cell destruction is far greater than erythropoiesis, with consequent anaemia.

Pregnancy and lactation increase the requirements of both folate and vitamin B_{12} in the same way as they do for iron. Hence megaloblastic anaemia more commonly occurs in pregnancy, especially in communities where marginal deficiencies exist. It is important that body stores of nutrients are made up after pregnancy because, if the diet is inadequate and a deficiency continues until the next pregnancy, the baby will be born with poor body stores. As we have seen such a continuing deficiency occurs with regard to iron, resulting in low haemoglobin values of cord blood, poor fetal stores of iron, and anaemia in infancy. Recovery of body stores of iron, folic acid and other nutrients may occur during school age, but body requirements increase again to sustain the growth spurt at adolescence. In many peasant communities early marriage and child-bearing is the rule, so that if a deficiency exists at adolescence it is transmitted to the offspring. Thus, in poor communities nutritional anaemia tends to be carried forward from one generation to another.

Folic acid deficiency also occurs in pre-term infants. Demands of growth exceed intake of the vitamin and they use up their tissue stores which, in any case, may be less than normal.

At birth serum and red cell folate levels are high in both pre- and full-term infants compared with adult values. They drop rapidly soon after birth in all infants, but the drop in value is more rapid and more severe in pre-term infants. The newborn infant's requirement for folate is 20 to 50 μg/l and most proprietary milks also provide the same amount. Warming the feeds after reconstitution for the purpose of sterilising will destroy the folate. For example, it has been shown that boiling for as little as 5 seconds reduces the folate content by 50 per cent. Folate deficiency should be suspected in all anaemic pre-term babies and particularly in those with very low birth-weights or those with a history of feeding difficulties.

In infants, repeated infections are known to cause anaemia with megaloblastic changes in the bone marrow. Similarly haemolysis due to any cause, e.g. malaria or sickle cell anaemia, increases the requirements of folic acid to meet the needs of a hyperactive marrow.

Megaloblastic anaemia due to deficiency of vitamin B_{12} is comparatively rare and is usually restricted to under-nourished communities who are on a predominantly vegetarian diet because of religious and cultural reasons. A megaloblastic anaemia caused by the fish tapeworm *Diphyllobothrium latum* is found in Finland and is due to a deficiency in the host caused by the tapeworm which diverts the vitamin in the gut lumen for its own use. In heavily infested areas of Finland, up to 27 per cent of the population are known to be carriers, and one in 50 such carriers is known to develop megaloblastic anaemia.

Loss of Nutrients

There are no physiological mechanisms for the excretion of iron except through the desquamation of cells lining the gut and of the skin. Hence the amount of iron in the body is mainly controlled by absorption.

The main cause of loss of iron from the body is through chronic blood loss — either from heavy periods or from the gut. In the tropics hookworm infestation is a well-known cause of iron deficiency anaemia. The adult worm is firmly attached to the mucosa of the gut and obtains blood from the host for its own needs of oxygen and glucose. Experiments with labelled iron in volunteers indicates that in heavy infections considerable quantities of blood may be lost (Table 1.21).

Table 1.21: Faecal Blood Losses Due to Intestinal Parasites

(ml/day)	Per parasite	Per 100 eggs in 1 g faeces
Necator Americanus	0.02–0.07	2.1
A.duodenale	0.14–0.26	4.4
Trichuris	0.005	0.25

In heavy infestations the losses cannot be recovered from the daily diet and over a period of time a debilitating chronic anaemia develops. As a general rule, above a critical load of 2,000 eggs of hookworm per g of faeces severe iron deficiency and anaemia are likely to occur.

Several cultural practices in traditional societies can contribute to iron deficiency through bleeding at periods when the body needs of iron are greatest. In several traditional societies of tropical Africa, the cutting of the uvula as a treatment for cough or for prophylaxis is a common practice. In many instances the procedure is carried out when the infant is three days old, and in some communities up to 96.2 per cent of infants have undergone the procedure before the age of six months. Similarly female circumcision is widely practised in tropical Africa. Blood loss at the time of the operation and the recurrent oozing of blood from the site may contribute to iron deficiency, especially if body stores are poor or during periods of rapid growth.

Where malaria is endemic it is a major cause of anaemia. Haemolytic anaemia is a common complication of pregnancy in Nigeria and responds to treatment with anti-malarial drugs and folic acid. It has been postulated that haemolysis in malaria is always in excess of the destruction of erythrocytes by the malarial parasites. This is because of an immunological response to malaria by the host. The body stores of iron, folic acid and other nutrients soon get exhausted because of an overactive marrow and because the poor diet supplies very little.

In addition to the direct effect on the erythrocytes, repeated malarial infection is also responsible for a chronic anaemia associated with enlarged spleen. In the so-called tropical splenomegaly syndrome, parasitaemia is scanty or absent and the red cell morphology resembles that of iron deficiency. Studies with labelled iron have shown a high plasma turnover of iron. A large number of erythrocytes are trapped in the enlarged spleen and represent a considerable portion of the red cell mass, which may be between 50 and 75 per cent of the total pool. It is likely that sequestration of such a large number of erythrocytes results in active erythropoiesis by the marrow, using up the available stores of iron and folic acid.

In conclusion, nutritional anaemias are the second largest group of nutritional disorders after protein-energy malnutrition. The individual is most vulnerable at those periods of life when the requirements for nutrients are increased because of the demands of growth. In many parts of the tropics, nutritional anaemia is particularly common on account of inadequate nutrition and super-added parasitic or helminthic infections, which further increase the requirements of nutrients. In many of the affluent societies of Western Europe, nutritional anaemia used to be a public health problem, not so very long ago. The present improvement is more due to better standards of health care, especially during infancy and pregnancy, and better nutrition, than to any public health measure.

Notes

1. The nine months of pregnancy are divided into three three-month periods of 'trimesters'.

References and Further Reading

Ebrahim, G.J., *Handbook of Tropical Paediatrics. Nutrition and Dietetics*, East African Literature Bureau, Nairobi, 1975.

Frood, J.D.L., Whitehead, R.G. and Coward, W.A., 'Relationship between pattern of infection and development of hypoalbuminaemia and hypo-β-lipoproteinaemia in rural Ugandan children', *Lancet,* 1971, vol. 2, p. 1047.

George, S., 'Food Aid? . . . or weapon?', *How the Other Half Dies,* Penguin Books, London, 1976.

Gopalan, C., 'Kwashiorkor and marasmus. Evolution and distinguishing features', in R.A. McCance and E.M. Widdowson (eds.), *Calorie Deficiency and Protein Deficiency,* J. & A. Churchill Ltd, London, 1968.

Holmes, A.M., Enoch, B.A., Taylor, J.L. and Jones, M.E., 'Occult rickets and osteomalacia amongst the Asian immigrant population', *Quart. J. Med.* 1973 NS XLII, 165, p. 1225.

McLaren, D.S., 'The great protein fiasco', *Lancet,* 1974, vol. 2, p. 93.

Mata, L.J., Kromal, R.A., Urrutia, J.J. and Garcia, B., 'Effect of infection on food intake and nutritional state: perspectives as viewed from the village', *Am. J. clin. Nutr.* 1977, vol. 30, p. 1215.

Morley, D.C., 'A health and weight chart for use in developing countries', *Trop. geogr. Med.* 1968, vol. 20, p. 101.

Morley, D.C., 'The severe measles of West Africa', *Proc. R. Soc. Med.* 1964, vol. 57, p. 846.

Olson, R.E. (ed.), *Protein-Calorie Malnutrition,* Academic Press, New York and London, 1975.

Oomen, H.A.P.C., McLaren, D.S. and Escapini, H., 'A global survey of xerophthalmia', *Trop. geogr. Med.* 1964, vol. 16, p. 271.

Rowland, M.G.M. and McCollum, J.P.K., 'Malnutrition and gastroenteritis in the Gambia', *Trans. roy. Soc. trop. Med. Hyg.* 1977, vol. 71, p. 199.

Rutishauser, I.H., 'The dietary background to protein-energy malnutrition in West Mango district, Uganda', in R. Owor, V.L.Ongom and B.G. Kirya, (eds.), *The Child in the African Environment,* East African Literature Bureau, Nairobi, 1975.

Shakir, A., 'The surveillance of protein-calorie malnutrition by simple and economical means' (a report to UNICEF), *J. Trop. Pediatr.* 1978, vol. 21, p. 69.

Tanphaichite, V. et. al., 'Clinical and biochemical studies of adult beri-beri', *Am. J. clin. Nutr.* 1970, vol. 23, p. 1017.

Venkataswamy, G., Krishnamurthy, K.A., Chandra, P., Kabis, S.A. and Pirie, A., 'A nutrition rehabilitation centre for children with xerophthalmia', *Lancet,* 1976, vol. 1, p. 1121.

2 THE PROBLEMS OF FOOD ABUNDANCE

R.J. Jarrett

For most people, an abundance of food is a relatively modern phenomenon — certainly when viewed against the whole of man's evolution and even in the context of recorded history. The abundance has coincided with industrialisation and the reduction in the expenditure of energy required for subsistence and transport. As a direct consequence of an increased availability of food energy and a decreased energy expenditure, obesity has become common and two associated diseases — atherosclerosis and diabetes mellitus — though not unknown before the eighteenth century, have become major causes of ill-health and of death. Heart disease secondary to atherosclerosis affecting the coronary arteries is now the single more common cause of death in industrialised societies. This chapter is concerned with the relation between food — both its quantity and quality — and these modern epidemics.

Obesity

'Let me have men about me that are fat' (Shakespeare. *Julius Caesar*)

'If to be fat be to be hated, then Pharaoh's lean kine are to be loved' (Shakespeare. *Henry IV*, Pt I)

'They are as sick that surfeit with too much as they that starve with nothing' (Shakespeare. *The Merchant of Venice*)

'Make less thy body hence, and more thy grace; Leave gormandising: know the grave doth gape for thee thrice wider than for other men' (Shakespeare. *Henry IV*, Pt II)

Thus Shakespeare expresses some of the attitudes — still prevalent — towards obesity. But what is obesity? How does one measure it? The term obesity is often used as a synonym for overweight, but the latter makes the assumption that, for a given height, there is a correct weight. However, people vary considerably in the contribution made to their total weight by their bones and their muscles. A few years ago a number of American football players were rejected for military service because they were 'overweight'. But when they were studied by physiologists who estimated their adipose tissue mass, they were found to have much *less* fat than men of apparently normal weight. There are a number of methods for measuring total body fat. These include the measured uptake of inert gases, e.g. cyclopropane or krypton, which are taken up specifically by adipose tissue, and densitometry by underwater weighing. These methods are all right for research but for clinical purposes measurement of subcutaneous fat at specific sites on the body, using special callipers, is more convenient, if less accurate. On average, about half of the body fat is subcutaneous. However, skinfold thicknesses must be measured with care — there is considerable observer variation in measurements made in the same people. Furthermore, body fat is distributed differently in individuals, in ethnic groups, by sex and by age, so that multiple measurements are more representative. The simplest method is to measure height and weight and express them as an index, the best one being the weight divided by the square of the height — sometimes known as Quetelet's Index. This is particularly useful for epidemiological indices where one requires to correlate 'obesity' with many other factors.

In assessing whether an individual is obese or not, use is often made of tables of height and weight which purport to give 'normal', 'standard', 'ideal' or 'desirable' weights. These are not satisfactory, for a number of reasons. Firstly, they are often based on unrepresentative populations and the circumstances of weighing and measuring — with or without clothes for instance — are often not known or not stated. Secondly, although some tables attempt to make allowances for different body builds, for instance by dividing people into small, medium and large frames, the definition of these is left to the discretion or imagination of the patient. Not unnaturally, people tend to choose their 'frame' to suit their weight! From the clinical point of view, therefore, obesity is best diagnosed by observation of the unclothed — or only partly clothed — body, supplemented if necessary by measurements of skinfold thickness.

The other deceptive feature of height/weight tables is that they obscure the effects of ageing. Thus there is no reason to suppose that the average increase in weight after growth has ceased should be regarded as normal in the physiological sense. Furthermore, as the author can testify, maintenance of the same weight after the age of 25 is often accompanied by transformation of muscle into fat tissue.

Some workers also make a distinction between types of obesity in relation to the distribution of fat. Simply but crudely there is a popular aphorism that fat accumulation is 'in men to tum and in

Figure 2.1: Gynoid and Android Obesity

a: Gynoid — or female-type — fat distribution in obese man and woman

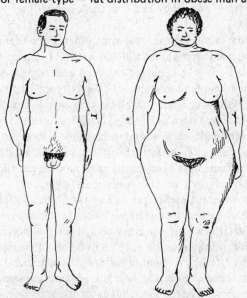

b: Android — or male-type — fat distribution in obese man and woman

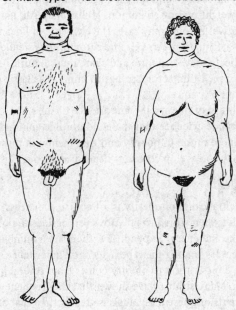

women to bum'. In more scientific, if less graphic terms, android
obesity is characterised by excess visible fat in the upper half of the
body and gynoid obesity by excess in the lower half (see Figure
2.1 a and b).

Apart from fat distribution, there are other differences in body
composition and shape which influence weight in relation to height.
Over the nearly three millennia of recorded medical history, there have
been several attempts to categorise man into 'types'. Hippocrates
(fifth century BC) recognised two 'temperaments' – phthistic and
apoplectic habitus. Galen's (129-199) classification into four types –
sanguine, phlegmatic, choleric and melancholic – based on the theory
of humours, dominated medical theory and practice until the
Renaissance. There have been several more modern classifications,
including Kretschmer's asthenic, athletic and pyknic types. However,
the best known, most useful, but still controversial, classification is that
of Sheldon, who devised a technique known as somatotyping. This was
based on the rating of three primary components – endomorphy,
mesomorphy and ectomorphy – on a seven point numerical scale.
Endomorphy rates the element of softness, roundness and smoothness,
but is not a measure of obesity, even though an extreme endomorph is
likely to be obese. Winston Churchill had a classic endomorph physique.
Mesomorphy rates bone and muscle development and the former
world heavyweight boxing champion, Muhammad Ali, may be taken
as representative. Ectomorphy rates the elements of linearity,
fragility and attenuation. An extreme ectomorph is slender, lanky, thin
and with delicate bone structure and spare musculature. Jacques Tati,
the famous French film actor, springs to mind as a classic example of
the ectomorph physique.

In the context of obesity the importance of the somatotypes is
that there is some evidence that the endomorphic and mesomorphic
physique is more prone to obesity and that men with these somatotypes
are more likely to develop coronary heart disease.

Causes of Obesity

The fundamental cause of obesity is, of course, an excess of food
energy which is then stored as fat. However, besides the obvious effects
of food intake and energy expenditure, there are a number of
permissive factors, among them being genetic inheritance. The evidence
for a genetic contribution to obesity comes from several kinds of
investigation. Many studies have shown that the frequency of obesity
amongst parents of obese individuals is greater than that amongst

parents of non-obese people. This might simply reflect shared habits, but it has also been shown that in families with natural and adopted children, only the weights of the natural children were significantly correlated with parental weights. More direct studies have been made upon identical and non-identical twins. Identical twins have a common genetic inheritance, so that differences between them must be predominantly environmental in origin. In one study of adult twins the mean difference in weight between identical twins was 4.1 pounds against 10 pounds for non-identical twins and 10.4 pounds for siblings of the same sex. Of course, this demonstrates similarity of weight and not necessarily of adiposity. However there are examples, both from man and other animals, of clearly inherited types of obesity. In mice, for instance, there is a much studied condition which is inherited as a recessive characteristic. This is the obese, hyperglycaemic syndrome which is characterised by extreme obesity, high levels of blood glucose and plasma insulin and a number of other metabolic and behavioural characteristics. In man there are several varieties of lipodystrophy, in which excessive amounts of fat are deposited in certain areas of the body, sometimes with virtual absence of fat in other areas. These conditions are rare, but it is a matter of common observation that some people deposit unsightly amounts of fat — for example around the ankles — without necessarily being particularly fat elsewhere. One remarkable ethnic variation of this local fat deposition occurs in the Kalahari Bushmen (Figure 2.2).

Nevertheless, most of the variation in adiposity is accounted for by other factors. The role of genetics is best expressed in Dobhzhansky's words 'what is inherited is not body weight as such, but the trend of the development of the body, which may result in different weights in different circumstances'. Or in other words, obesity is a product both of nature and of nurture.

Cultural Factors

Kelly West, who has studied a wide variety of populations of differing races, religions and cultures, has remarked upon the degree with which environmental factors may influence adiposity in groups with a similar genetic background. In poor communities in Asia and Central America, obesity was very rare. However, above a certain level of economic attainment, other factors began to operate. In Uruguay, for example, he found that urban people were much fatter than their rural counterparts even though their racial origins and their income levels were similar.

Figure 2.2: Ethnic Steatopygia (excessive fat in the buttocks) in a
Female Bushman (this is confined to women and is also known as
'Hottentot bottom')

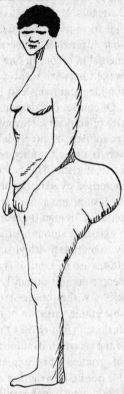

A remarkable example of culturally determined obesity – and of the
effects of overnutrition – was that described by one of the intrepid
Victoran explorers of Africa, J.H. Speke. In his book 'Journal of the
Discovery of the Source of the Nile' he describes his visit to the Kingdom
of Karagwe

> . . . after a long and amusing conversation with Rumarika in the
> morning, I called on one of his sisters-in-law. She was another of
> those wonders of obesity, unable to stand excepting on all fours. I
> was desirous to obtain a good view of her and actually to measure
> her . . . After getting her to sidle and wiggle in the middle of the
> hut, I took her dimensions: round arm 1 foot 11 inches; chest

4 ft 4 inches; thigh 2 ft 7 inches; calf 1 ft 8 inches; height
5 ft 8 inches. All of these were exact except the height, and I
believe I could have obtained this more accurately if I could have
laid her on the floor. Not knowing what difficulties I should have to
contend with in such a piece of engineering, I tried to get her height
by raising her up. This after infinite exertions on the part of both
of us was accomplished, when she sank down again fainting. Mean-
while her daughter, a lass of sixteen, sat stark naked before us,
sucking at a milk pot, on which the father kept her at work with a
rod in his hand, for as fattening is the first duty of a fashionable
female life, it must be duly enforced by the rod, if necessary.

A less extreme example of a culturally determined obesity is the
Japanese sumo wrestler. Sumo is an ancient sport dating back 1500
years and is the national sport of Japan. Trainees usually enter the
wrestler society — currently about 800 strong — in their late teens. The
majority become overweight and obese despite their strenuous
training because their special diet contains about twice as many calories
as that of the Japanese average. A group of 96 wrestlers, whose average
daily consumption exceeded 5000 kilocalories was recently compared
with a control group; they had significantly elevated blood pressure,
triglyceride and uric acid levels, all factors which tend to be higher in
the obese. However, not all the wrestlers were obese. Judged by body
density measurements 53.4 per cent were both 'overweight' and
obese while 39.1 per cent were 'overweight' but not obese. The
remainder were of 'normal' weight.

The fact that many of these wrestlers were not obese despite a large
calorie intake is an indication of the importance of exercise in weight
control. Traditionally, boxers training for their fighting weight lose
their excess pounds by physical exercise rather than food restriction.
The amount of energy used in some activities is surprisingly (to some)
great and is, in general, proportional to the weight of the participant.
According to the American nutritionist Mayer, who is a principal
advocate of the role of activity in weight control, the increase of
energy expenditure per hour over energy used in sitting is, for the
'average man' — 100-550 kcalories for walking (varying with the speed),
up to 585 kcalories for cycling, up to 685 kcalories for swimming
and skating and up to 950 kcalories for skiing or climbing.

The fact that an overweight individual must use more energy to
perform the same amount of exercise than someone of normal weight
has an important secondary consequence. Thus if a physically active

individual increases his energy intake and puts on some weight, the extra energy cost of performing his usual physical activity will tend to reduce his weight again, so achieving a new balance.

Dietary surveys of population samples, both of adults and of children, have shown an inverse relationship between total calorie consumption and the degree of obesity — measured either by skinfold thickness and/or by indices of height/weight. In other words, fatter people tend to eat less than thinner people. At first sight this is surprising; however, the missing measurement is the corresponding degree of activity. There are several studies in which activity has been measured and related to the degree of obesity. These have included direct observation and indirect measurements using a device which records the heart rate and gives an integrated (average) rate over a defined period. Within certain limits, heart rate is related to activity. Both types of study have shown that obese people, in general, are less active than people of normal weight. In a study of high-school girls in Massachusetts, Mayer and Johnson examined both the dietary intake and exercise patterns. The obese girls were matched for age and height with non-obese and were found to separate into two groups. The larger of these included girls who ate slightly less than the normal weight girls, but who exercised considerably less, with 'sitting' activities, like watching television, emphasised at the expense of walking and active sports. This association of fatness and inactivity may start very early in life — perhaps one expression of the genetic contribution to obesity. Mayer, with another collaborator, Rose, studied babies aged 4 to 6 months. Fatness was not related to food intake, nor growth to food intake, but there was a high degree of positive correlation between physical activity, food intake and slimness. So fat babies had small to moderate intakes, but were very inactive.

Mayer illustrates the lack of physical activity possible in modern civilisation with a parable of the modern American male which serves for many other countries too:

> he gets up, and, after briefly standing in front of his mirror using his electric toothbrush and his electric razor, sits down at the breakfast table, goes on to sit in his car, in his office, at coffee break, at lunch, in his office, in his car, at dinner, and in front of the television set; and, after lying in a warm bath for a while, goes on to lie in a bed. Should he (or his wife) be briefly disturbed during the evening meal or when he is already in bed by the ring of the telephone, extensions have been placed in his house to prevent his

having to stir himself.

In case anyone should think that physical inactivity is a purely American phenomenon, let me quote the British physiologist, Passmore:

> ... it is not generally recognised how sedentary is the life led by most urban people. Even young military cadets spend 17¾ hours a day either lying, sitting, or standing; the corresponding figure for coal miners is 18¾ hours a day and for colliery clerks, 20 hours a day. Military cadets and miners have two of the most physically active occupations, and yet about three-quarters of their life is sedentary.

Thus weight control both in the short term and particularly over a lifetime is a balance of the amount and nature of food intake and the amount and nature of physical activity. This fact is one which both individuals and communities must face, for there is good evidence that obesity is still increasing in frequency even in those countries which have been relatively affluent for several generations.

The Cost of Obesity

The more extreme obesity carries with it a number of obvious penalties. Thus clothes often have to be specially made and are anyway hard to get. Fat women often have to resort to clothes designed for expectant mothers. Overlapping folds of fat create conditions – hot and moist – for fungal infections of the skin, which cause irritation and a nasty smell. Getting in and out of vehicles – or chairs – can be difficult and running for a bus or train is even more so. The breathing difficulties of the very obese have a number of components, one being mechanical interference with breathing due to the presence of fat in and around the respiratory muscles. This sometimes leads to retention of carbon dioxide – due to poor ventilation – and consequent somnolence, giving rise to the Pickwickian syndrome, so-called because of the character 'fat Joe' in Pickwick Papers ... ' – and on the box sat a fat and red-faced boy, in a state of somnolency, whom no speculative observer could have regarded for an instant without setting down as the official dispenser of the contents of the before-mentioned hamper, when the proper time for their consumption should arrive'.

Presumably because they tend to be slow and ungainly, obese people are prone to accidents of all kinds – in the home, at work, and in the street.

Prolonged obesity may eventually lead to mechanical disabilities.

Anatomists say that man is still not adequately adapted to the erect posture — even when lean — and carrying permanently an extra, heavy load is mechanically undesirable. The consequences include degenerative arthritis, particularly of hips, knees and lumbar spine. Furthermore, in an elderly person already handicapped by a stroke, a fracture or by arthritis, concomitant obesity makes rehabilitation more difficult. Because the abdominal muscles are rendered less effective by the presence of fat, abdominal hernias are more common in the obese. This abdominal fat also makes obese people unpopular with surgeons who have to operate upon them. It makes the operation technically more difficult and local complications — such as wound infection — are more common. Post-operatively, the complication of venous thrombosis and pulmonary embolism (blockage of a pulmonary artery) is also more likely to occur. At least one surgical procedure is more common in the obese — operations on the gall bladder, for gall stones are more frequent.

Adult onset diabetes mellitus is more common in the obese and this will be discussed more fully later in this chapter.

However, most of the discussion about the cost of obesity centres round its effect upon life expectancy. Statistics from American insurance companies loom large in this discussion. Tables 2.1 and 2.2 are taken from the data presented by the Metropolitan Life Insurance Company and are based upon approximately five million policy holders in the United States and Canada. They are the basis for the practice of insurance companies of charging higher life insurance premiums for overweight people. As discussed earlier these data relate to weight and not specifically to adiposity.

Table 2.1: Mortality Among Overweight Persons

| | Excess mortality (%) | | | |
| | 10% or more above average weight | | 20% or more above average weight | |
Age	Men	Women	Men	Women
15–39	17	14	31	21
40–69	21	23	31	32

Source: Metropolitan Life Insurance Company, Build and Blood Pressure Study, 1960

Table 2.2: Causes of Death with Excess Mortality Among Overweight
Men and Women

Cause of death	Excess mortality (%)	
	Men	Women
Diabetes mellitus	133	83
Ischaemic heart disease	35	35
Vascular lesions of the central nervous system	53	29
Pneumonia and influenza	32	27
Diseases of the digestive system	68	39
Accidents and homicides	18	—

Source: Metropolitan Life Insurance Company, Build and Blood Pressure Study,
1960

Of the listed causes of death in Table 2.2, the single most important
one is ischaemic heart disease. This is a common cause of death in the
population as a whole, so a given percentage increase in risk affects a
lot of people in terms of absolute numbers. The relationship of obesity
to disease and death from coronary heart disease has aroused much
controversy, which has been resolved, at least in the opinion of many
observers, by the results of several prospective studies of population
groups. In these studies a number of measurements were made at a
baseline examination and these have been subsequently related, using
sophisticated and complex statistical methods, to the observed
episodes of coronary heart disease. In general, the results have shown
that obesity — whether measured as relative weight, as fat fold
thickness or as a weight/height index — is a risk factor (or more
precisely, a risk index) for coronary heart disease. However, obesity is
significantly correlated with blood pressure and serum cholesterol levels
and when these are considered, together with obesity, in the risk index
equation, obesity per se does *not* appear as an index of risk. The
usual interpretation of these analyses is that the added risk associated
with obesity is due to the 'complications' of obesity, namely high levels
of serum cholesterol and blood pressure. A further complication,
diabetes mellitus, also increases the risk of coronary heart disease,
though, in terms of the *whole* community, obese or not, its contribution
is relatively small.

The only manifestation of coronary heart disease which can be
linked directly with obesity is angina pectoris (pain in the chest on
exertion). This is presumably because for a given amount of exercise an

obese person will expend more energy than a thin one and, therefore, increases more the workload of the heart. If the coronary circulation is similarly impaired, angina will, therefore, be more likely to occur in the obese.

Coronary Heart Disease

This is the premier epidemic of modern times and has become the commonest single cause of death in nearly all countries sufficiently affluent to produce statistics on mortality (Table 2.3). Its rise is the principal reason why the expectation of life of a man age 40 has not increased since the beginning of this century — despite all the apparatus of modern medicine. It was not unknown before this century: indeed, Heberden described the syndrome of angina pectoris in 1768.[1] However, it was not until the 1920s that the differentiation between angina pectoris and myocardial infarction (death of cardiac muscle secondary to interruption of its blood supply — often called, though not strictly correctly, coronary thrombosis) became widely known and part of the apparent increase in coronary heart disease is due to more accurate diagnosis. Nevertheless, in many parts of the world today coronary heart disease is a rare condition. The populations with a low frequency are usually poor, rural communities operating a subsistence economy. One well known exception to this is Japan, where until fairly recently, coronary heart disease was very uncommon.

If coronary heart disease were simply a cause of death after the Biblical three score years and ten, it would not be regarded as a problem. However, it is a significant cause of death in the middle-aged and, if less than 40 years be young, increasingly so in the young as well. In the United Kingdom in 1973, for instance, 52 per cent of all deaths in men aged 45-54 years were due to cardiovascular disease and more than three-quarters of these were due to coronary heart disease. In this age group, women are less affected — 28 per cent of deaths were due to cardiovascular causes and under half of these were due to coronary heart disease. In men aged 35-44 years, 41 per cent of deaths were due to cardiovascular disease and about three-quarters of these were due to coronary heart disease. It is in this age group that the most rapid increase in the death rate from coronary heart disease has occurred in recent years (Table 2.4). It has been calculated that if all coronary heart disease could be prevented, the average life span for a British male would increase by 7 years and for a British female by 9 years. This contrasts with the effect of a cancer cure, which would only add about two and a half years to the average life expectation of both sexes.

Table 2.3: Deaths from Ischaemic Heart Disease per 100,000 in the Age Group 45-54 years in 1970

Country	Men	Women
Finland	403	55
USA	346	83
Scotland	343	81
Australia	297	77
New Zealand	273	18
Canada	270	48
England and Wales	259	42
Norway	213	23
Netherlands	201	25
Czechoslovakia	194	38
Israel	194	59
Federal German Republic	148	26
Hungary	146	38
Sweden	137	25
Italy	106	21
Bulgaria	72	26
France	66	12
Romania	61	20
Spain	50	10
Hong Kong	34	12
Japan	34	14

Source: WHO Statistics Annual

The factors involved in the increase in coronary heart disease are complex; but there is no doubt that changed patterns of nutrition are important. Most of the communities where coronary heart disease is rare live (or till recently lived) upon diets which are high in carbohydrate (cereals, grain, vegetables) and low in fat, in particular saturated fat. Animal protein is often, but not always, also a restricted item of diet. In communities where coronary heart disease is common, the proportion of calories from carbohydrate and fat is similar. Furthermore, much of the carbohydrate is taken in the form of sugar and much of the fat is saturated.

Most observers think that the most important change has been towards a higher proportion of fat in the diet and to the greater proportion of saturated fat, the effect of this being to raise the prevailing levels of serum cholesterol, which is one of the major risk indices of coronary heart disease within communities. In international comparative studies, the distribution of serum cholesterol levels has also been the main discriminating measurement between communities with high and low frequencies of coronary heart disease. There is a great deal of experimental work which supports the view that an elevated serum cholesterol level is not an epiphenomenon,[2] but a direct cause of the lesions in the walls of the arteries (known as atheroma or atherosclerosis) which by promoting thrombosis or by directly causing obstruction are responsible for the clinical manifestations. The role of serum cholesterol is strikingly, though tragically, demonstrated in those rare individuals who inherit the condition known as familial hypercholesterolaemia (receiving one gene from each parent) and who have very high serum cholesterol levels at birth. These unfortunate people develop severe atherosclerosis in childhood and adolescence and die from coronary heart disease, usually before the age of twenty-five. Although animal models of atherosclerosis are admittedly unsatisfactory in terms of the human disease, it is possible to produce considerable elevation of serum cholesterol levels and subsequent arterial wall lesions by feeding animals diets high in cholesterol and saturated fat.

Table 2.4: Annual Death Rates per 100,000 from Coronary Heart Disease for Men and Women Aged 35-64 Years in England and Wales

| | Age | | | | | |
| | 35—44 | | 45—54 | | 55—64 | |
	Men	Women	Men	Women	Men	Women
1950–52	33	8	167	42	566	211
1960–62	53	8	217	39	655	194
1970–72	66	10	274	46	717	194
1973	64	11	286	52	731	205

Nevertheless, some workers have put forward the view that it is sugar, not fat, which is the principal dietary factor responsible for coronary heart disease. It is certainly true that there is a high correlation between the consumption of sugar and fat within populations. But, in the individual, it is much easier to alter serum cholesterol levels by changing fat consumption than by altering sucrose consumption; and in experimental animals, atherogenic diets based on fat are more effective than those based on sucrose.

It is also argued that man is adapted to eating animal fat, because, as a hunter he has always consumed animals. However, this argument fails to take account of the qualitative changes in the kind of animals consumed now compared with those eaten by our forebears. Wild animals are lean, with little subcutaneous fat and even less within their muscles. Contrast this with the meat from the domesticated sheep, cattle and pigs which we eat today. Even the leanest steak is 'marbled' with fat. Furthermore the nature of the fatty acids in the fat has changed. Animals living on woodland and bush vegetation, which is rich in oil and which is typical of pre-agricultural vegetation, have a high percentage of polyunsaturated fatty acids in their body fat. Animals living on water-rich grassland, which includes some present-day wild animals as well as domesticated animals, normally wild animals kept in zoos, and man himself, have a much smaller proportion of poly-unsaturated fatty acids. So, whatever diet man is adapted to, it is certainly not one high in saturated fats; nor, of course, one high in sucrose.

One of the recurrent challenges to those who believe in the 'fat' hypothesis of atherogenesis is the experience of several groups of nomads in Somalia, Kenya and Tanzania where diet is said to consist mainly of milk, meat and blood. Despite this apparently atherogenic diet, they have low serum cholesterol levels and little, if any, coronary heart disease. They are lean and active people, with relatively low blood pressure levels, which do not rise with age. Further, it seems that their food intake is irregular and they intersperse periods of plenty with periods of starvation. A recent observation concerning milk may also help to explain their low cholesterol levels. In an experiment in Cambridge, people were given diets which included four pints of milk daily, one group consuming whole milk and another group consuming skimmed milk (i.e. with the cream removed). The experiment only lasted two weeks, but in both groups there was a significant fall in serum cholesterol, much greater in the skimmed milk group, where the fall was from a mean of 200 mg/100 ml to 188 mg/100 ml. In another group given butter yielding the same amount of fat and cholesterol as the 4 pints of whole milk, the mean cholesterol level rose, as expected. So it is possible that whole milk and skimmed milk, but not butter, contains a factor which actually lowers the serum cholesterol. Claims have been made that such a factor has been isolated and partially characterised.

One method of studying the effect of environment as compared with heredity is to look at people who have migrated from one country to another. There have been several such studies in relation to coronary heart disease, the most rigorous one being of Japanese immigrants into the United States, mostly into California. The immigration occurred mainly in the late nineteenth and early twentieth centuries. There was a much higher death rate from coronary heart disease in the Japanese Americans compared with Japanese in their native land, though a lesser one from strokes. That this was not due to different practices in certification was confirmed by post-mortem examinations and by a comparison in the living of the frequency of angina pectoris and of abnormalities of the electrocardiogram, both of which were more common in the Japanese Americans. The major differences observed in blood biochemistry were higher average serum cholesterol, glucose, uric acid and triglyceride concentrations in the Japanese Americans. Blood pressure levels were not different. This kind of study illustrates the importance of environmental factors in the causation of coronary heart disease, even if it does not tell us precisely what those factors are.

One of these factors may be associated with the constituents of the water supply. There is a strong statistical association between cardiovascular mortality and the mineral content of drinking water (see Tables 2.5 and 2.6), which has been found in many countries, though not in all investigations. The association is not with any one kind of cardiovascular disease and different varieties are associated with the water supply in different countries. In England and Wales, where the most intensive studies have been carried out, the correlation is strongest between mortality rates and water calcium and carbonates. Despite a great deal of research, however, it is still not known how the association comes about. Presumably it must be a mechanism common to the several varieties of cardiovascular disease, and blood pressure could be such a common factor. The role of trace elements, like cadmium, manganese, chromium and vanadium, is also being studied. Recently, it was suggested that the water factor might be silicon. This element is mainly found in connective tissue and particularly in the arterial wall, being concerned in the architecture and strength of connective tissue and membranes. Silicon levels are reduced in atherosclerotic arteries. It is by no means proven that lack of silicon contributes to atherosclerosis, but it is an attractive hypothesis, which should stimulate further research. It also neatly links the water story and the fibre story, which will be discussed later. In brief, a reduction in the amount of fibre is characteristic of the diet of industrialised societies. As fibre is a rich source of silicon, it is at least possible that a low fibre intake leads to a relative silicon deficiency.

Table 2.5: Some of the Countries Reporting an Association Between Cardiovascular Mortality and Water Components

Country	Type of cardiovascular disease
Japan	Cerebrovascular
Sweden	Cerebrovascular (women); 'Degenerative' heart disease
USA	All varieties: but predominantly hypertensive heart disease
England and Wales	All varieties
Holland	Coronary heart disease in women
Canada	Coronary heart disease
Finland	All varieties
Australia	Coronary heart disease; cerebrovascular disease
Ireland	All varieties

Table 2.6: Mean Death Rates per 100,000 in the Years 1958-64 from Cardiovascular Disease in the ages 45-64 in the 61 County Boroughs of England and Wales with a Total Population Exceeding 80,000 in 1961

Water calcium (parts per million)	Number of towns	Men	Women
10	8	751	355
10–39	24	721	330
40–69	9	636	306
70–99	13	633	281
100+	7	546	248

Before leaving the subject of nutrition and coronary heart disease it must be emphasised that there are many factors concerned in the genesis of atherosclerosis and also in the production of cardiac abnormalities (see Table 2.7). Furthermore, as there is little evidence to suggest that in developed countries the *amount* of atheroma has increased much in the

Table 2.7: Some of the Factors Shown to be Associated Statistically with the Frequency of Coronary Heart Disease

---

Age
Blood groups other than O
Cholesterol level in blood
Chromium deficiency
Climate
Coagulation disorders
Diabetes
Education
Family history
Fat intake
Haematocrit values
Heart rate at rest
High blood pressure
Obesity
Personality type
Sex (i.e. gender)
Smoking
Stress
Sugar intake
Triglyceride level in blood
Uric acid level in blood
Water constituents

---

past 50 years, a period during which there has been a large increase in coronary heart disease *deaths*, there may well be factors which are not concerned in the genesis of atherosclerosis but which do affect the response of the cardiac muscle to an impaired blood supply. Some of these factors may well be nutritional — like the water factor(s) — while others, like cigarette smoking, are environmental, but not nutritional. Prospective studies in the United States, Sweden and the United Kingdom have shown that the factors which are the most powerful predictors of future coronary heart disease are age, the levels of serum cholesterol and blood pressure, and the number of cigarettes smoked. Cholesterol is present in several distinct lipoproteins in plasma and the level of cholesterol in the high density lipoprotein fraction is *inversely* related to subsequent coronary heart disease and there is biochemical evidence that this lipoprotein may have a protective, anti-atherogenic role. Apart from age and cigarette smoking, all the factors mentioned can be modified by the nature of the diet.

Diabetes Mellitus

This is a very ancient disease, referred to in ancient Hindu and Egyptian writings. The best known classical description is that of Aretaeus (120-200 AD), the Cappadocian physician:

> Diabetes is a wonderful affection, not very frequent among men, being a melting down of the flesh and limbs into urine. Its cause is of a cold and humid nature, as in dropsy. The course is the common one, namely, the kidneys and the bladder; for the patients never stop making water, but the flow is incessant, as if from the opening of aqueducts. The nature of the disease, then, is chronic, and it takes a long period to form; but the patient is short lived, if the constitution of the disease be completely established; for the melting is rapid, the death speedy. Moreover, life is disgusting and painful; thirst unquenchable, excessive drinking, which, however, is disproportionate to the large quantity of urine, for more urine is passed; and one cannot stop them either from drinking or making water. Or if for a time they abstain from drinking, their mouth becomes parched and their body dry; the viscera seem as if scorched up; they are affected with nausea, restlessness, and a burning thirst; and at no distant term they expire.

However, this classical form of diabetes mellitus, which reaches its peak incidence in early adolescence, is not caused by nutritional lack or excess and is nowadays overshadowed by the much more frequent kind of diabetes, known as maturity-onset diabetes because it usually appears after the age of forty. The major differentiating factor between the two types of diabetes is that the classical diabetic is absolutely dependent upon an external supply of the pancreatic hormone insulin. Without it he will become ill and will die within days, weeks or, occasionally, months. The maturity-onset diabetic, however, can usually be controlled by dietary manipulation, sometimes with the aid of anti-diabetic drugs, occasionally with the aid of insulin. However, insulin here is used as an expedient, not as an absolute necessity. It has recently been demonstrated that there are other differences between the two types of diabetes. Thus, there is an association between insulin-dependent (usually young-onset) diabetes and certain of the antigens (rather like the well known blood-group antigens on the red cells) found on the white cells of the blood and known as the histoincompatibility antigens. There is also an association between insulin-dependent diabetes and several conditions thought to be caused by auto-immunity (see chapter 3), such as certain thyroid gland disorders, pernicious anaemia and hypofunction of the adrenal cortex (Addison's Disease). Notwithstanding these differences, both types of diabetic are prone to complications which affect the eyes, the kidneys, and the peripheral and autonomic nervous systems. Diabetics, at least in most communities, are also more likely to develop atheroma and, secondary to this, coronary heart disease, cerebro-vascular disease and peripheral vascular disease. In general, these complications are related to the duration of the diabetes, though many diabetics of long standing, for reasons which are unknown, nevertheless escape any significant ill-effects of the disease.

Maturity-onset diabetes has been increasing in frequency in most countries. Part of this increase is spurious, due to technological improvements in biochemical tests upon blood and urine, to a greater awareness of the disease and even to specific attempts to screen communities for diabetics. Nevertheless, there is good evidence of an increase in North America and Western Europe and, in certain population groups, there has been an explosive epidemic of diabetes. The two most outstanding examples of this are the Pima Indians of Arizona and the inhabitants of Nauru, a small island in the Central Pacific.

The Pima Indians and their ancestors have lived in the Arizona desert for two thousand years, cultivating crops with the help of water from the Gila River. For many years their health care has been in the hands of the Indian Medical Service and it would appear that diabetes was an uncommon condition before the Second World War. In 1963 it was noted that many of the adult Pima had diabetes and in 1965 a systematic study of diabetes was begun. It was subsequently found that diabetes was extraordinarily frequent – with about half of those aged 45 years and above having the disease. This was a typical maturity-onset kind of diabetes, with all the usual complications, except the atherosclerotic ones.

Nauru has several claims to fame. It is the smallest republic in the world and its inhabitants have the highest per capita income in the world – thanks to the fact that most of the surface of Nauru contains high-grade phosphate ore. The Nauruans have also been systematically studied and a prevalence of diabetes as high – or even higher – than that amongst the Pima discovered.

Both the Pima Indians and the Nauruans have radically changed their mode of life in the past few decades. One of the consequences of these changes is that both groups have become very obese. In the Pima the average energy intake is over 3000 kcalories and in Nauru it is over 6000! The major items in the Pima diet are pinto beans, tortillas made from wheat flour and chilli peppers. They eat less sucrose than the general population of the United States, but about the same proportion of saturated and unsaturated fats. Nevertheless, the average serum cholesterol level is relatively low — below 200 mg/100 ml — and coronary heart disease is uncommon in diabetics as well as non-diabetics, though slightly more frequent in the diabetics. However, they do have a high frequency of gall-stones and gall-bladder disease, possibly due to an increased excretion of cholesterol into the bile.

While it is uncertain whether obesity can account for all of the excess of diabetes in the Pima and Nauruans, there is no doubt that adiposity is an important factor in predisposition to maturity-onset diabetes. This has been clearly demonstrated in studies within countries by comparing newly diagnosed diabetics with control groups matched for age and sex. Furthermore, even in non-diabetics the level of blood sugar after an oral glucose load[3] is related to the degree of adiposity. Perhaps the most striking demonstration of the effects of adiposity was made by two Americans — West and Kalbfleisch — who investigated comparable population samples in a number of countries and were able to estimate the prevalence of diabetes in each (Table 2.8). They found an enormous difference between the lowest and highest frequencies and when they looked for possibly related factors, they found that the highest degree of correlation was between the frequency of diabetes in each population and the corresponding frequency of obesity. There was a poorer correlation with average calorie intake and no discernible relationship with the *kind* of food consumed.

The Pima and the Nauruans are not the only people who have experienced an explosive increase in the frequency of diabetes. Several other North American Indian tribes, groups of Polynesians, Asian Indians in South Africa and Australian Aboriginals have all been similarly affected. This mid- to late-twentieth-century phenomenon affecting people emerging from subsistence economies has led the American geneticist, Neel, to propose his 'thrifty gene' hypothesis. Neel suggested that subjects from populations which had been subjected to fluctuations of food supplies and who might have experienced periods of abundance alternating with periods of famine, might have developed a propensity to store food as adipose tissue in times of abundance and, at the same time maintain normal blood sugar levels. This trait might offer selective advantages for survival during a period of famine, in which case it would become common throughout the population by genetic selection. Given perpetual 'abundance', however, the trait is disadvantageous, leading to obesity and thence to diabetes. While the theory is obviously untestable, it is a plausible explanation of the observed phenomena. There are parallels in the animal world. Certain desert animals – the Egyptian sand-rat, the Chinese hamster, the tuco-tuco – when transferred to a laboratory or a zoo and fed a standard diet tend to develop diabetes.

Table 2.8: Frequency of Diabetes Mellitus in Samples Above the Age of 34 Years in Seven Populations

East Pakistan (now Bangladesh)	2.0%
Malaya (now Malaysia)	3.3%
Central America	4.1%
Uruguay	6.9%
Venezuela	7.0%
United States	15.0%
Cherokee Indians in North Carolina	25.0%

Source: K.M. West and J.M. Kalbfleisch, 'Diabetes in Central America', *Diabetes,* (1970), vol. 19, p. 656.

Not all maturity-onset diabetes is secondary to obesity – an appreciable number of lean persons develop typical maturity-onset diabetes. In developing countries, diabetes may actually be caused by *under-nutrition.* One variety appears to be due to protein deficiency during growth, causing pancreatic calcification, and is seen in tropical areas of Africa and India, in particular where cassava is the staple cereal. Also in India, in the tribes of Southern India, people who are very undernourished throughout life, diabetes is not uncommon.

The place of diet in causing diabetes has been debated for many years. In the 1930s, Himsworth collected data on food consumption and diabetes mortality rates from many countries and came to the conclusion that the highest diabetes rates occurred in those countries with relatively high fat and low carbohydrate diets. He adduced experimental support for this by demonstrating that a reduced carbo-hydrate intake led to impaired glucose tolerance – measured by the blood glucose response to an oral or intravenous glucose load. The fat hypothesis has been challenged by a number of workers, in particular Yudkin, who has shown that fat and sucrose consumption within countries is highly correlated. Yudkin has also claimed that, when national diabetes mortality rates in the mid-1950s are related to average national sugar and fat intakes about twenty years earlier, there is a better correlation with sugar intake than with fat intake. Cleave has put forward a hypothesis suggesting that a large number of diseases are predominantly caused by the change to high consumption of refined carbohydrate, predominantly sucrose, and that diabetes is one of these conditions. The evidence is largely epidemiological in nature, based upon rates of diabetes in population groups which have changed their dietary habits. The most widely quoted example is that of the Yemenite Jews who had emigrated to Israel. It was observed that the frequency of diabetes in newly-arrived immigrants was very low – of the order of 0.06 per cent. In similar immigrants, settled in the country for twenty-five years or more, the frequency was 2.6 per cent, a forty-fold difference, presumably due to environmental factors. It was claimed by Cohen and his colleagues, who carried out the study, that the major change in dietary habits was an increase in sucrose consumption and that this was the cause of the increased frequency of diabetes.

The problem of evaluating studies of this kind is that many changes accompany 'acculturation', amongst them being, usually, an increase in the frequency of obesity, which in most studies is the most impressive correlate of diabetes frequency. Another Israeli study provides more direct evidence against sucrose being a specifically diabetogenic factor. In a large prospective study of Israeli Civil Servants, dietary information was collected on individuals prior to the development of diabetes. Those who ultimately developed diabetes during the period of observation actually consumed *less* sugar on average than those who remained non-diabetics. The confounding factors are again obesity and energy expenditure, for, as mentioned earlier in this chapter, on average fat people eat less of all energy containing foods than thin people.

My own interpretation of the available evidence is that the principal environmental factor in the causation of diabetes is adiposity. The determinants of this will vary between different cultures and between individuals in the same culture. Also the influence of a given degree of adiposity will depend upon the genetic constitution of the individual as well as upon other, less well defined, factors.

Nutrition and the Consequences of Diabetes

Although the evidence is incomplete, there does not seem to be much difference in the frequency of the more specific, microvascular complications of diabetes[4] in different ethnic groups, with widely different nutritional habits. However, the frequency of disease of the larger arteries, secondary to atherosclerosis, does differ widely between diabetics in different populations and approximately parallels the frequency in the corresponding populations of non-diabetics. Thus the frequency is low in diabetics in countries where the overall frequency is also low — and vice-versa. In Japan coronary heart disease as a cause of death in diabetics was only about one fifth as frequent as in the United States, though about twice as common as in non-diabetics in Japan. As mentioned earlier, this is not an ethnic characteristic, for Japanese migrants to the United States have rates of coronary heart disease similar to that of the other citizens. It does suggest that environmental factors are important; the striking dietary differences between the traditional Japanese and the modern American diet life in the amount and kind of fat and the amount of complex carbohydrate consumed.

Hypertension

In recent years it has become possible to record the arterial blood pressure continuously and these measurements have shown considerable variation throughout the day, with the blood pressure falling to (previously) surprisingly low levels during sleep. However, most of the information we have about raised blood pressure and its consequences comes from 'casual' measurements.

The level of blood pressure in an individual depends upon a number of factors. There is a genetic component, demonstrated by studies on twins, siblings and families. There are also a number of environmental factors. Exercise, cold and anxiety raise the blood pressure acutely. Adiposity is positively correlated with blood pressure and this is independent of the difficulty in measuring the blood pressure with the conventional cuff sphygmomanometer in a fat arm. In all industrialised communities where surveys have been made there is also an average rise of blood pressure with age. However, there have been a number of studies in primitive societies where average blood pressures have been the same across the age range. These include the African Bushmen (see Introduction), several Pacific Island communities and East African nomads. Men from the latter group serving in the Kenyan army showed a rise in blood pressure levels after some years, suggesting that their blood pressure pattern is determined by environmental factors and is not an ethnic peculiarity.

The environmental factor most studied is salt intake. It has been known for a long time that drastic salt restriction can lower the blood pressure even in people with severe hypertension. Furthermore, in animal experiments it has been possible to raise the blood pressure by feeding increased amounts of salt. The increase did not occur in all animals and it was possible to breed strains of rat particularly sensitive to the effects of salt. It is likely, but not certain, that the situation in man is similar; the evidence is indirect. Thus in certain communities — South African blacks and certain Japanese fishing communities — hypertension is common and salt intake high. However, studies in the United States and in Britain have failed to find any relationship between salt intake and blood pressure. The situation may be similar to that of dietary fat and plasma cholesterol levels. Thus, above a certain threshold of salt intake genetic factors may be principal determinants of blood pressure level in the individual.

Blood pressure levels are very important as determinants of disease. Again insurance company statistics have demonstrated the risks. The American Society of Actuaries published data from the experience of 26 American insurance companies between 1935 and 1954. Both men and, though to a lesser extent, women with raised blood pressure levels suffered a significantly diminished expectation of life. Thus a man aged 45 with a systolic blood pressure of 150 mm/Hg and a diastolic pressure[5] of 100 had an expectation of life eleven years less than a man with pressures of 120 and 80 respectively. The two most important causes of death attributable to hypertension are heart disease and strokes. Although strokes are relatively more common in people with hypertension it is the generally more common heart disease which accounts for most of the excess premature deaths. Most of the heart disease is secondary to coronary artery disease, but high blood pressure can also cause heart failure by the chronic increase in the workload of the left ventricle in expelling blood into a high pressure system. The insurance data have been amply confirmed by prospective population studies like that at Framingham, Massachusetts. These have also confirmed the observation that the extra risk is graded, that is, there is no sudden threshold of blood pressure level above which a risk becomes evident.

Alcohol

Alcohol in excess can produce psychological and physical dependence as well as, more directly, a number of physical ill effects. Psychological dependence upon alcohol – alcoholism – is difficult to define exactly and many definitions exist, the most cynical being that which defines an alcoholic as 'someone who drinks more than his doctor'.[6] A more useful definition is 'an alcoholic is a person who cannot stop drinking when there is good reason for doing so'. The good reason may be an illness secondary to alcohol consumption or a marital or employment problem engendered by alcohol.

There are several forms of alcohol abuse. Regular – but restrained – dependence is seen particularly in people whose job is such that regular drinking is convenient or necessary. Such people do not have a 'problem' – unless they are required to give up drinking, or until it becomes necessary to start drinking earlier and earlier in the day, or until they develop a physical illness due to the alcohol.

A compulsive addict drinks until his supplies are exhausted or until he is helpless. Unable to control the quantity he drinks, he is often obviously intoxicated. This is the form of alcoholism often portrayed in films and books and not a few writers have succumbed themselves. Yet another variety is the periodic drinker, someone who indulges in bouts of excessive drinking – the lost weekend – and who may be a social drinker otherwise.

Physical symptoms are not prominent in the pre-addictive stage. They include loss of memory for a previous night's drinking and gastric irritation. Psychological symptoms include anxiety and depression. These may have contributed to the reason for drinking in the first place, but they are often made worse by the alcohol.

The organ most often damaged by alcohol is the liver, not because it is peculiarly sensitive, but because it is the most active organ in metabolising alcohol. Some 70-80 per cent of all alcohol metabolism takes place in the liver and, when excessive, the chemistry of the liver cell is deranged, with subsequent damage to its structure. One of the biochemical abnormalities, probably under-recognised, is alcoholic hypoglycaemia (low blood sugar). This usually occurs after a drinking bout, particularly if it occurs after several days of poor food intake, allowing liver glycogen[7] stores to become depleted. Hypoglycaemia, if profound, leads to a state of coma or semi-coma which may be diagnosed as alcoholic intoxication. It is more dangerous, however, and can be fatal or may lead to irreversible brain damage.

In heavy drinkers the liver almost always becomes infiltrated with fat, a process which is reversible and in itself not a cause of serious disturbance. Alcoholic hepatitis (liver cell damage) does not usually occur before 10 years or more of heavy drinking. With abstinence, combined with a high calorie, high protein diet, recovery can sometimes occur, but the mortality rate remains high. Those who recover are at risk of developing cirrhosis of the liver later. Cirrhosis is a diagnosis based upon the pathological appearance of the liver and includes a fibrous tissue reaction, with disruption of the liver's lobular pattern, regeneration in a nodular pattern and vascular derangement.

It has been estimated that of all the cases of cirrhosis in the world at least 50 per cent are linked to alcohol abuse. In the United Kingdom there are at least 1500 deaths per year from cirrhosis and in the United States it ranks seventh in the all-cause death list. In France, where liver disease and cirrhosis are very common, studies have shown that above a threshold alcohol consumption of 60 g per day in men and 20 g per day in women the morbidity from cirrhosis increases steadily with increasing consumption, an increase which is exponential in nature.

Cirrhosis can not only lead to liver failure directly, it also predisposes to tumour formation. If this occurs, then the downhill course to liver failure and death is accelerated.

Alcohol Intake and Cancer

Apart from cancer of the liver, alcohol intake is also associated with cancer of the mouth, pharynx, larynx and oesophagus. In Europe, for instance, the highest frequency of oesophageal cancer is found in Brittany and Normandy, where consumption of cider and cider-based liqueurs is high. There appears to be an interaction between the alcohol intake and cigarette smoking, but how this comes about is still a mystery. One suggestion is that an agent which is soluble in alcohol — but not in water — may be responsible for initiating the cancer.

Other Effects of Alcohol

There is little doubt that the effects of alcohol upon the central nervous system are responsible for many road accidents and also for a proportion of criminal activity. Addiction to alcohol is responsible for much marital unhappiness and for problems at work. In fact, alcoholism is much more likely to present itself to a doctor in the guise of marital problems, work difficulties, a history of aggressive behaviour, financial embarrassment and trouble with the law, rather than as a physical illness.

The psychological and neurological effects of alcohol excess may be acute, as in alcoholic intoxication. They may also occur after brief abstinence from alcohol and include tremulousness, auditory hallucinations, epilepsy, delirium tremens and delusional states. There are also a number of disorders of the nervous system which occur in chronic alcoholism which seem to be due, in part, to absolute or relative deficiency of B vitamins. Finally, suicide is very much more common amongst alcoholics and alcoholism seems to be particularly associated with suicide amongst doctors.

The heart is also directly affected by alcohol. The condition known as alcoholic cardiomyopathy has been described in many countries, both rich and poor. It usually presents as an arrhythmia,[8] less often as heart failure. In the absence of other causes, a long history of high alcohol consumption is suggestive. Alcohol seems to have a direct deleterious effect upon the heart muscle and the microscopic abnormalities seen in man have been reproduced in experimental animals fed on ethanol, beer or wine.

In 1973 a further effect of alcohol was noted as the 'fetal alcohol syndrome'. Children of alcoholic mothers were observed to have a characteristic facial appearance, poor growth before and after birth, delayed central nervous system development, with and without mental deficiency, and an increased frequency of congenital anomalies, such as cleft palate and heart lesions. This syndrome, at least in part, usually occurs in the infants born to women who are chronically heavy drinkers, but also in women who are 'binge' drinkers and who only drink socially between bouts. That alcohol itself is the causative factor has been confirmed by experiments in animals.

Nutrition and Cancer

The frequency of specific cancers varies greatly both from place to place and from time to time, largely due to the effects of environmental factors. The most striking example is that of carcinoma of the bronchus which, over the past fifty years has increased in frequency to become the commonest fatal cancer in men in Britain. In other parts of the world, for instance parts of Africa, it is still fairly uncommon. The possible role of nutritional factors in causing cancer is strongest for cancers of the oesophagus, stomach, liver and colon.

There are a few areas where cancer of the oesophagus is very common. These include the Ghurjev region of Kazakhstan on the north

coast of the Caspian, black Africans in the Transkei and in Bulawayo
and the Honan province of China. Where studies have been made a
relationship has been found between the frequency of the cancer and
both alcohol consumption and cigarette smoking, though these two
factors alone do not account for the very high frequency in certain
areas.

Cancer of the stomach is common in Eastern Europe, Japan,
Iceland and Chile, but is declining in frequency in most countries. The
differences in frequency cut across racial lines, the blacks in the United
States having a higher frequency than the whites, whereas all European
countries have higher frequencies than black Africa. It seems likely
that there are carcinogenic factors in some simple diets, but there is
little evidence to suggest what they are — or were.

As discussed earlier, cancer of the liver may occur as a result of
cirrhosis secondary to excessive alcohol intake. In the tropics there is
another, much commoner, cause of liver disease and cancer. Some years
ago there was an outbreak of poisoning which killed 100,000 turkeys
in British farms. This was traced to a consignment of peanut meal
contaminated with the fungus Aspergillus flavus which produces a
toxin — aflatoxin. This was later found to produce acute liver failure in
poultry and, when given in very small doses, cancer of the liver in a
wide variety of animals. It is known that human liver cells contain the
enzymes necessary to produce the metabolites of aflatoxin which are
the actual carcinogens. The fungus frequently contaminates foodstuffs
stored under hot and humid conditions — as in the tropics — and it
has been demonstrated that in several countries the frequency of liver
cancer is related to the amount of aflatoxin consumed in the diet.

Cancer of the colon is also related to culture rather than race. In the
United States the frequency is similar in whites and blacks. In Hawaii
it is equally common in Caucasians, Japanese and Hawaiians; it is rare
in Japan itself and in Africa. In general it is common in industrialised
populations, but even there considerable differences in frequency occur
within and between countries. Several aspects of diet may explain
these geographical differences. It has, for instance, been postulated
that a high fat diet increases the concentration of bile acids in the large
bowel, with subsequent conversion by bacteria to substances which are
directly carcinogenic or co-carcinogenic. Meat consumption is
strongly correlated in international comparisons with colon cancer
frequency. Although, in theory, amino-acids could be metabolised to
carcinogens or co-carcinogens, no direct evidence has so far been
obtained. A currently fashionable hypothesis relates to the other feature

of modern diet, its depletion of fibre, and is discussed in the section on dietary fibre.

Another factor which is attracting increasing attention in relation to cancer is the intake of nitrates. The main sources of these are vegetables and drinking water, with cured meat products such as bacon and sausages also contributing. The theoretical basis of the suspicion of nitrates is that they can be converted by bacterial action and by acidic stomach contents to N-nitroso compounds, which are potent carcinogens in all laboratory animals tested. There is evidence that populations consuming large amounts of nitrate tend to have high mortality rates from stomach cancer and nitrate consumption has also been linked with cancer of the oesophagus, kidney and liver. The nitrate levels in drinking water are increasing in many places because of the widespread use of nitrates as fertilisers and much more information is needed to determine safe levels of nitrates in drinking water so that policies on fertiliser use can be rationalised.

Dietary Fibre

Once every 10 years or so a new idea emerges about the cause of disease that captures the imagination and, for a time, seems to provide a key to the understanding of many of these diseases whose aetiology was previously unknown. Such ideas have included the concepts of hormone deficiency and excess, inborn errors of metabolism, vitamin deficiency, septic foci, psychosomatic disease, stress and auto-immunity. To these we may now add a deficiency of dietary fibre. But whether it will be as seminal an idea as that of vitamin deficiency or as sterile as that of stress, we shall probably not know for another 10 years.[9]

There is a great deal of current interest and speculation and an increasing amount of research concerning the role of dietary fibre in the cause of disease. While the concepts are not new the fact that they are now widely discussed is largely due to three people. The first of these, Surgeon Captain Cleave, was impressed by the changes in the diet of industrialised countries and by the concomitant change in the patterns of disease. Furthermore, he observed that diseases now common in industrialised societies were not so in the underdeveloped countries. He argued on evolutionary grounds that these new diseases must be due to a failure to adapt to new factors in the environment and that dietary changes were the most important ones. He was impressed by the increasing refinement and processing of food which led to a high consumption of starch in general and sucrose in particular. The argument is set out in more detail in the latest edition of Cleave's monograph.[10]

Burkitt and Trowell,[11] drawing upon their extensive experience of rural Africa, have modified Cleave's theory. They suggest that the ill-effects of over-refining food are due not so much to excess *consumption* but to a deficiency of a necessary element in man's diet — fibre. On epidemiological grounds, mainly the absence or rarity of such conditions as diabetes, obesity, atherosclerosis and non-infective bowel diseases such as diverticulosis, adenomatous polyposis, cancer and ulcerative colitis, in rural populations of developing countries, they suggest that fibre deficiency is a major cause of a wide variety of disorders.

The simplicity of this theory is very attractive, particularly to those who share the current disillusion with modern technology. Conversely, its universality antagonises many scientists who have a basic distrust of all-embracing theories of disease aetiology. And it must be admitted that some protagonists of the hypothesis antagonise by their very fervour.

Fibre and its Sources

The term 'dietary fibre' is not very precise. Literally, it includes nerve and muscle fibres as well as plant fibre and non-absorbable foodstuffs such as pectins, gums, lignins and hemicellulose, which are not fibrous in nature. Spiller has suggested the term 'plantix' to include all plant fibre plus other non-digestible plant carbohydrates, but this new word has yet to become generally acceptable and I shall therefore use 'dietary fibre' in this account, implying non-absorbable food constituents.

The principal sources of dietary fibre are cereals, starchy roots, tubers, fruit and, in certain countries, unrefined legumes. Wheat, which is the major cereal in many countries, is milled to various degrees of extraction. Wholemeal (or wholewheat) flour is 100 per cent extraction and is milled by grinding the whole of the wheat kernel. The flour is naturally brown in colour (unlike much brown bread which is so because of added colour) and is rich in crude fibre. In Britain, however, over 90 per cent of flour used is white (70 per cent extraction) and has a low fibre content. Oatmeal, rolled oats and rye flour are richer in fibre than low extraction wheat flour.

Maize (corn) is another common cereal and the source of a number of proprietary breakfast foods — which are usually low in fibre, being prepared from low extraction flour. In rural Africa, however, maize is consumed simply pounded as whole grain or as a lightly milled maize meal.

In Asia, the traditional cereal is rice, much of which is only lightly processed and, therefore, rich in fibre.

The fibre-rich starchy roots, tubers and fruit include potatoes, yams, cassava, sweet potatoes, dates and dried figs. The fibre-rich legumes include several varieties of beans and peas.

A fall in fibre consumption has occurred in industrialised communities over the past 100-150 years principally because of changes in the extraction rate of wheat flour and also because of a reduction in the amount of bread eaten. In Britain, for instance, in the mid-nineteenth century the average consumption of bread was about 600 g per day and the bread was made from lightly-milled wheat grain which would contain a substantial amount of fibre. Today the average Briton eats only about 200 g of bread each day and the bread is made from low extraction flour with a much lower fibre content.

The Consequences of Fibre-Depletion

There are several diseases which are rare in rural areas of under-developed countries, in particular rural Africa, but which are common in industrialised countries and becoming more common in those inhabitants of rural areas who become urbanised. A case can be made for many of these conditions resulting, at least in part, from changes in the fibre content of the diet. Table 2.9 indicates those considered by Burkitt and Trowell[12] to have the strongest claim to be due to fibre deficiency. I propose now to consider the evidence in the individual conditions, excluding obesity, diabetes, and ischaemic heart disease, which have been considered earlier and whose relationship with fibre deficiency is very tenuous.

Dental Caries

Dental caries and periodontal disease is common amongst both children and adults in industrialised countries, but it was not always so, as studies on teeth and jaws of skulls of neolithic man and subsequently have shown. Further, the pattern of dental caries has also changed. It is now common for caries to start near the point of contact of adjacent teeth, but in ancient peoples it usually started near the margin of the gums. The frequency of caries and periodontal disease increases rapidly in a population becoming urbanised.

Table 2.9: Diseases and Disorders Postulated to Result from the Consumption of Fibre-Depleted Foods

---

a) Related to the gastrointestinal tract
   constipation
   appendicitis
   diverticular disease
   hiatus hernia
   colonic cancer
   polyps
   haemorrhoids
   dental caries
b) Miscellaneous
   obesity
   diabetes mellitus
   ischaemic heart disease
   gall stones

The usual explanation for this has been the increased consumption of refined carbohydrate, in particular, sucrose. These foodstuffs promote the formation of dental 'plaque', which consists of densely packed colonies of bacteria (Streptococcus mutans appears to be the principal bacterium involved) in an adherent film of gelatinous materials. This plaque can directly affect the teeth or may cause inflammation of the periodontal tissues. The effect of plaque on the teeth also depends on the degree of host resistance, which can be increased by fluoride administration during the time of tooth formation. However, there is good evidence that the composition of the diet in other respects also affects the tissue. Experimental studies have demonstrated the presence of protective factors in unrefined foods and vigorous mastication — necessary with fibrous foods — may enhance their effect. Vigorous mastication may also be beneficial in other ways — by promoting saliva flow, thus 'flushing' the teeth and buffering the acidity of the dental plaque — and by causing wear and flattening of the cusps of the teeth: this would reduce the depths of the fissures and thus areas of potential food stagnation. In other words a fibrous diet automatically carries out those measures of dental hygiene which we perform (or should perform) with a toothbrush.

Bowel Mobility and Diseases of the Large Bowel

In man the colon (large bowel) has several functions, including the conservation of certain of its contents (bile acids; water) and as a reservoir. Absorption of water converts the fluid effluent of the small bowel into the solid or semi-solid stool. The process is aided by the movements of the colon – the circular muscle contracting and slowing the onward movements of the faeces, producing a segmented colon. Vegetable and cereal fibres adsorb water and thereby increase the bulk of the faeces in the colon. Bulky faeces have two effects upon the colon – they increase the rate of passage of the faeces and they tend to diminish the pressures within the lumen. High fibre diets also increase the rate of transit through the small bowel.

The effect of faecal bulk upon transit time and the bulking effect of cereal and vegetable fibre has been used for a long time in the treatment of constipation. It was known to the 'Father of Medicine' Hippocrates who, in 430 BC wrote 'to the human body it makes a great difference whether the bread be made of fine flour or coarse, whether of wheat with the bran, or without the bran' and 'wholemeal bread clears out the gut and passes through as excrement'. A Persian physician, Hakim, made a similar observation about chupatties in the ninth century AD. When wheat bran is added to a typical modern diet the usual effect is a softening of the faeces and an increase in its weight. However, it used to be thought that bran, along with undigested vegetable residues, would 'irritate' the colon and this concept gave rise to the term 'roughage' to describe high fibre containing diets. This view – a purely armchair conception and never based on direct evidence – has been disproved and in fact reversed, for high fibre diets are now used, with some success, in the treatment of people with 'irritable' bowels – people with a functional disturbance of the bowel usually known today as 'the irritable bowel syndrome' – as well as those with organic/functional disorders such as diverticular disease. Probably the main beneficial effect in these conditions is secondary to the bulkier, softer nature of the faeces which require less muscular effort on the part of the circular muscle of the colon to carry out its normal segmenting action.

The amount of faeces passed each day varies considerably in different cultures, averaging 100-150 g on a typical modern 'Western' diet and nearly 500 g in rural Africans eating a traditional high cereal/ high fibre diet. Comparative average transit times from mouth to anus – measured by ingesting radio-opaque pellets – are approximately 80 hours and 35 hours respectively. All these average figures, of course, conceal a great deal of individual variation.

Diverticular Disease of the Colon

Diverticulae of the colon are small, saccular outpouchings of the mucous lining membrane through the investing muscle layer. In themselves they are harmless, but they may become the site of inflammation — diverticulitis — which may involve the tissues outside the bowel and lead to peritonitis. Although diverticulae and diverticulitis were described in the early nineteenth century they were regarded as rarities. They appear to have become very much more common during the first two decades of the present century and now about 5 per cent of those over 40 and over one-third of those over 60 years of age have diverticulae — though diverticulitis itself is much less common. The frequency of diverticulae has similarly increased with urbanisation of rural communities in Africa and elsewhere.

In view of the known physiology of the colon — outlined above — there seems a good *a priori* case for incriminating the decline of fibre as the main causative agent in the rise of diverticular disease. Increased pressures in the colon over long periods of time — as mentioned above it is a disease of late middle-age and later — may reasonably be expected to cause the extrusion of the mucous membrane. Furthermore, the relief of symptoms commonly experienced when a bulkier stool is induced by cereal or vegetable fibre also offers support to the theory. This relief has now been demonstrated in properly controlled trials, though we do not yet know whether the treatment will prevent the complication of diverticulitis in someone who already has diverticulae.

Appendicitis

This too is a common condition which was rare in the nineteenth century. Although, in 1827, it was suggested that abscesses in the lower right abdomen were secondary to perforation of the appendix, the condition was still referred to as 'perityphlitis'. The term 'appendicitis' did not become popular until the late nineteenth century. In Britain and in the white population of the USA there was a rapid increase in the frequency of appendicitis during the first two decades of the twentieth century, but the rise did not occur until much later in the black American population. Today the frequency is identical in both white and black populations. Unlike diverticular disease, a noticeable rise in the frequency of appendicitis has been seen shortly after a change to a low fibre diet. Thus African soldiers normally accustomed to a traditional diet and given European-type diets on military service have experienced a rapid rise in the frequency of appendicitis.

The appendix normally fills and empties during the processes of digestion and it is suggested that the changed consistency of the faeces on a low fibre diet is more likely to lead to obstruction of the appendix. In particular the occurrence of faecaliths — hard, stone-like bodies, which do not ordinarily form in soft faeces — predisposes to obstruction. Obstruction leads to appendicular colic and, if unrelieved, to mucosal damage and inflammation. Again, this theory is not definitely proven, but it is a plausible explanation of the observed phenomena and no other satisfactory explanation exists to challenge it.

Tumours of the Large Bowel

Both benign and malignant tumours of the large bowel are rare in undeveloped communities. In industrialised communities, however, cancer of the large bowel is one of the most common forms of cancer — along with cancer of the lung or breast. Not much is known of the history of cancer of the large bowel, but studies in developing countries and of migrants from areas of low to those of high incidence leave little doubt that environmental factors are important in its genesis. However, even between countries with similar economic development there are large variations in incidence. Thus the mortality rate for cancers of the colon and rectum is two and one half times greater in Scotland than in Norway. So it seems likely that the environmental factors concerned are complex. Indeed, five nutritional theories have been proposed to explain the differences — (a) amount of animal protein (b) increase in sucrose (c) increase in refined food (d) amount of fat (e) fibre depletion. Much of the evidence for each of these theories is epidemiological, based on comparisons of average intake of various foods in areas of high and low incidence. There has also been experimental work analysing the chemical and microbiological characteristics of faeces from these areas and differences have been found in the concentration of bile acids and sterols and in the prevailing kinds of bacteria. It has been suggested that a high fat diet predisposes to higher levels of bile acids and sterols and that the kinds of bacteria predominating in faeces from areas of high cancer incidence may degrade sterols to potentially carcinogenic substances. The concentration of bile acids and sterols can be diminished in the faeces by decreasing fat intake or by increasing fibre intake and the fibre protagonists have suggested that the latter is the more important fact, both in terms of international differences and as a possible means of prevention.

A recent comparison of a high incidence area in Denmark with a low incidence area in Finland suggests that the situation may be more complex than the above model. The major dietary differences were a ninefold excess of beer consumption in Denmark and a fourfold excess of milk drinking in Finland. The Danish subjects also consumed significantly more white bread, meat, wine and spirits and less potatoes and less dietary fibre. However, intestinal transit times were similar as were the concentrations of faecal steroids. In another comparison of Hawaiian Japanese and indigenous Japanese, who have very different risks of colon cancer, there was also no difference in intestinal transit time; though stool weights were significantly higher in the indigenous Japanese.

Hiatus Hernia

The oesophagus passes through a gap or 'hiatus' in the diaphragm to reach the stomach. Ordinarily the stomach remains in the abdomen, but sometimes it herniates into the chest through the hiatus – hence 'hiatus hernia'. There are two main types. The less common is paraoesophageal, where part of the stomach herniates up beside the oesophagus. The more common is the sliding hernia, where the oesophago-gastric junction slides up through the hiatus. Not all herniae give rise to symptoms. The symptom usually associated is dyspepsia, in particular a burning sensation behind the sternum due to reflux of acid gastric contents into the oesophagus. Hiatus hernia is a disorder of late middle age and above, is much more common in women and is often associated with obesity, gall stones and diverticular disease.

The epidemiology of hiatus hernia is very difficult to determine. It can only be confidently diagnosed by radiology and the frequency of diagnosis depends on the technique used and on the radiologist's criteria. Nevertheless the frequency is probably low in undeveloped countries.

The thesis that fibre deficiency is concerned in the genesis of hiatus hernia is purely speculative. It is assumed that movement of the stomach into the chest is due to raised pressure in the abdomen and that a fibre-depleted diet leads to intermittently raised abdominal pressures during straining at stool. As yet there is neither direct nor indirect evidence to support the hypothesis.

Venous Disorders

Varicose veins and haemorrhoids are very common disorders of developed countries and thrombosis in veins — not necessarily varicose — is also a fairly common cause of illness and a not uncommon cause of death when the clot breaks off and blocks the pulmonary artery or one of its major branches (pulmonary embolism). Like diverticular disease, these venous disorders are much less common in undeveloped communities, but increase in frequency with urbanisation. Precise comparisons are difficult because there is no universal standard for diagnosing either varicose veins or haemorrhoids, particularly the minor degrees of abnormality.

Theories concerning the genesis of varicose veins and haemorrhoids have generally invoked increased pressure in the usually low pressure venous system. The venous disorders often first appear or are exacerbated during pregnancy and may subside afterwards, suggesting that the pressures exerted by the gravid uterus may be important. Raised pressure within the abdomen, whether caused by the pregnant uterus or by straining at stool, is transmitted to the veins in the leg if the valves within the veins become incompetent. These valves normally prevent peripheral flow in the veins, flow towards the heart being induced by the pumping action of the leg muscles. It is suggested that repeated, intermittent raised abdominal pressure during defaecation results, in predisposed individuals, in incompetence of the valves and subsequent venous dilatation and varicosity.

Another factor which might contribute to venous disorders in the legs is the position adopted during defaecation. The traditional position is squatting, which compresses the veins in the legs and protects them against any rise in intra-abdominal pressure. It is also possible that the muscular effort involved in defaecation is less in the squatting position than in the sitting position on the raised toilet, which would imply that intra-abdominal pressures would be lower.

Cleave has argued that another predisposing factor is pressure by a loaded colon on the iliac veins. This has led to some dispute amongst surgeons and anatomists as to whether a loaded colon would, in fact, have such an effect and must be regarded as *sub judice*. All the arguments put forward above are, of course, largely hypothetical but they do appear to be consistent with what is known of venous anatomy and physiology.

So far as the haemorrhoidal veins are concerned, they are largely unprotected from a rise in intra-abdominal pressure. Existing piles are made worse by straining at stool so it is not unreasonable to suppose that it is also the major factor in the genesis of piles.

Dietary Goals for Industrialised Countries

Readers of the two preceding sections might well be able to construct a list of desirable changes in national food habits likely to promote health. A similar task has been undertaken by the US Senate Select Committee on Nutrition and Human Needs[13] whose chairman, Senator George McGovern stated 'the eating patterns of this century represent as critical a public health concern as any now before us. We must acknowledge and recognise that the public is confused about what to eat to maximise health . . . We have an obligation to provide practical guides to the individual consumer as well as set national goals'. The advice the committee actually gave was broadly similar to that contained in Scandinavian recommendations for a healthy diet[14] and set out six dietary goals as well as guidelines, mostly relating to the prevention of coronary heart disease, from various expert and official bodies.

The six goals were:

(1) To increase carbohydrate consumption to between 55 and 60 per cent of the total energy intake. The increase should be in the form of complex carbohydrates, such as vegetables, fruits and whole grains which would also contain other nutrients, including fibre.

(2) To reduce fat consumption to no more than 30 per cent of total energy intake (N.B. while this is less than the proportion of fat in the British diet during World War 2, it is more than that usual in traditional Mediterranean cooking).

(3) To alter the nature of dietary fat. Saturated fats to be reduced to 10 per cent of total energy, balanced against 10 per cent mono-unsaturated and 10 per cent polyunsaturated fats. (This compares with the current British average of 21 per cent saturated, 16 per cent mono-unsaturated and 4 per cent poly-unsaturated = total 41 per cent of dietary energy.)

(4) To reduce dietary cholesterol to 300 mg/day.

(5) To reduce refined sugar to 15 per cent of dietary energy (compared with the current British average of 20 per cent).

(6) To reduce salt intake to approximately 3 g/day.

The committee noted that highly processed foods are most likely to be high in saturated fat, sugar or salt — and also contain nutritionally unnecessary additives such as artificial colouring. In the United States, in particular, soft drinks have become a major source of sucrose.

Very few, if any, nutritionists would quarrel with these goals, though some would emphasise one rather than another or would perhaps dispute the exact goal figures. Evidence that the more highly educated members of society are gradually adopting these goals into their life style is accumulating from a number of studies. However, there is tremendous commercial pressure towards consumption of confectionery, alcoholic beverages and highly processed foods — witness television and other advertising and the layout of the average supermarket — and it seems unlikely that the mass of the population will adopt these goals unless governments do more than exhort. It is possible to modify choices and behaviour by fiscal measures. For instance, the relative consumption of butter and margarine in Britain has varied greatly over the past ten years or so. Butter consumption increased when its price was subsidised in May 1973 and again when subsidies were increased in 1974 and 1975. Consumption dropped in 1976 when subsidies were twice reduced substantially. The subsidy was temporarily suspended at the end of 1976 and in the early part of 1977 sales of butter fell steeply. The sales of margarine went up on each occasion as the sale of butter declined. In both Britain and the USA over the past ten years there has been a decline in the average intake of eggs and animal fat and a rise in the consumption of vegetable fats and oils. Whether this is due to economic factors or to deliberate changes in life style as a result of health consciousness is largely unknown. There is, of course, within the food industry a great deal of advertising on behalf of the special margarines high in unsaturated fats, which may also be having an effect upon consumer choice.

These changes in food consumption together with a decline in cigarette consumption have been accompanied by a fall in mortality from coronary heart disease, firstly in the USA and more recently in Britain. Although we cannot know for certain, only a determined sceptic would deny the possibility — if not the probability — that the changes in consumer habits have produced the changes in mortality.

Notes

1. Heberden's original description did not relate the chest pain to the heart. It seems to have been Edward Jenner — of smallpox inoculation fame — who first made the connection — 'it was suggested by Dr Jenner that the angina pectoris arose from some morbid change in the structure of the heart, which change was probably ossification, or some similar disease, of the coronary arteries'. C.H. Parry, *An Inquiry into the symptoms and causes of the Syncope Anginosa, commonly called Angina Pectoris, illustrated by dissections,* Bath and

London, R. Crutwell, 1799.

2. Communities in which the levels of cholesterol are high also tend to be well supplied with television sets and motor cars. But if these do contribute to coronary heart disease it is in a much less direct way.

3. The so-called glucose tolerance test is often used as a diagnostic test for diabetes mellitus. There are various tests which differ in detail, though the principle is the same. A glucose load is given after a period of fasting, usually overnight, and may be given either by mouth or as an infusion into a vein. The blood glucose level is measured before administering the load and at various intervals afterwards.

4. In particular disease of the small blood vessels (capillaries) in the retina, the light sensitive tissue at the back of the eye.

5. The blood pressure varies with the contraction and relaxation of the left ventricle which expels blood into the arterial system. The systolic blood pressure is the highest and the diastolic pressure the lowest in each cycle.

6. Unfortunately, this definition may be too strict, for doctors are one of the high risk groups for alcoholism.

7. Glycogen is the storage form of glucose and is present in liver and muscle. Liver glycogen is readily broken down to glucose which is discharged into the blood stream. In the fasting state this is the mechanism which maintains the normal level of blood glucose.

8. A disorder of the normal rhythm of the heart, which may be experienced by the individual as palpitations.

9. R. Doll, in *Refined Carbohydrate Foods and Disease*, D.P. Burkitt and H.C. Trowell (eds.), (Academic Press, London, New York, San Francisco, 1975).

10. T.L. Cleave, *The Saccharine Disease* (Wright, Bristol, 1974).

11. See D.P. Burkitt and H.C. Trowell (eds.), *Refined carbohydrate foods and disease: some implications of dietary fibre* (Academic Press, London, New York and San Francisco, 1975).

12. Ibid.

13. 'Dietary goals for the United States', US Senate Committee for Nutrition and Human Needs (Washington D.C., 1977).

14. See S. Davidson, R. Passmore, J.F. Brock and A.S. Truswell (eds.), *Human Nutrition and Dietetics* (Edinburgh, 1975), p. 652; Royal Norwegian Ministry of Agriculture Report, no. 32, to the Storting (1975–6) on Norwegian nutrition and food policy (Oslo).

References and Further Reading

Burkitt, D.P. and Trowell, H.C. (eds.), *Refined Carbohydrate Foods and Disease: some implications of dietary fibre,* Academic Press, London, New York and San Francisco, 1975.

Cleave, T.L., *The Saccharine Disease,* Wright, Bristol, 1974.

Davidson, S., Passmore, R., Brock, J.F. and Truswell, A.S. (eds.), *Human Nutrition and Dietetics* (6th edn), Churchill Livingstone, Edinburgh, London and New York, 1975.

Dobhzhansky, T., *Mankind Evolving,* Yale University Press, New Haven, 1962.

Doll, Richard, *Prevention of Cancer. Pointers from Epidemiology,* Rock Carling Fellowship, Nuffield Provincial Hospitals Trust, 1967.

Edwards, G. and Grant, M., *Alcoholism: new knowledge and new responses,* Croom Helm, London, 1977.

Kannel, W.B., McGee, D. and Gordon, T., 'A General Cardiovascular Risk Profile: The Framingham Study', *American Journal of Cardiology*, vol. 38, 1976, pp. 46–51.

Mayer, J., *Human Nutrition: its physiological, medical and social aspects*, Charles C. Thomas, Springfield, 1972.

West, Kelly M., 'Diabetes in American Indians and Other Native Populations of the New World', *Diabetes*, vol. 23, 1974, pp. 841–55.

3 NUTRITION AND IMMUNITY

R.N. Poston

1. Introduction

The object of this chapter will be to discuss and clarify the role of the immune response in relation to nutrition. This relationship is of three kinds: nutrition can affect immune responses; dietary proteins can evoke immune responses; and immune responses can impair nutrition.

The defects of the immune system in malnutrition may be the problems with the greatest social importance in the field of immunology today. This is because the impairment of the immune defences is a major factor in the high incidence of infectious disease in under-developed countries, and study of this defect may contribute to the management of this enormous problem. Malnutrition is largely a paediatric problem in these countries, and its deleterious effect on immunity highlights the importance of breast feeding in the maturation of the immune system.

Food and the bacterial contents of the gut act as a continual source of immune challenge to the body. A specialised part of the immune system exists in the gut to meet this challenge, but abnormalities in the immune response induced can occur. These can lead to damage of the gut and other tissues by a variety of hyper-sensitivity mechanisms, producing such diseases as malabsorption and food allergy.

Firstly in this chapter, the basic nature of the immune system will be outlined, bearing in mind that some readers may be unfamiliar with immunology. Then particular attention will be given to the relationship of the immune system and the gut which, in part, has only recently been discovered. After these preliminaries, I hope the reader will not be completely baffled by the intricacies of the complex interactions of diet, cells and antibodies that follow.

2. Basic Immunology

The keys to the understanding of the immune system lie in the lymphocyte and the nature and consequences of the interaction of antigen and antibody.

Lymphocytes

All lymphocytes are ultimately derived from bone marrow stem (precursor) cells. Some migrate eventually to the lymph nodes and spleen and differentiate; as a consequence their surface membrane bears immunoglobulin, which they have synthesised in small quantity. These are called B lymphocytes (B for bone marrow, or, conveniently, Bursa of Fabricius, a lymphoid organ adjoining the cloaca in birds, essential in them for the development of these cells; no mammalian equivalent of the bursa has been found). B lymphocytes (B cells), which are recognisable experimentally by detection of their surface immunoglobulin, are capable of further differentiation and division to become antibody-secreting plasma cells. One lymphocyte and its progeny of plasma cells can synthesise only one specific antibody, i.e. one that will react with a particular foreign substance, an antigen. It seems that lymphocytes are produced capable of manufacturing immunoglobulins with millions of different antibody specificities; this is probably controlled genetically, but the exact mechanism for the generation of this diversity remains controversial. However they originally came into being, it is known that lymphocytes are stimulated to divide and produce many daughter lymphocytes and plasma cells on exposure to the antigen with which their particular antibody reacts. Antibodies formed by plasma cell secretion appear in the blood plasma. The daughter lymphocytes are long lived, and by their presence the body becomes sensitised to an antigen to which it has been previously exposed. A primary antibody response on first exposure to an antigen is comparatively slow and small. In a secondary response to subsequent exposure, the 'memory' lymphocytes can respond rapidly by division and differentiation to plasma cells, so the response is quicker and larger.

Another population of lymphocyte precursors migrates from the bone marrow to the thymus, where the cells divide and mature into thymus-dependent or T lymphocytes (T cells). These disseminate through the body early in life and join the B cells in populating the spleen and lymph nodes. They do not synthesise antibody, but despite this can become sensitised to antigens and give rise to a progeny of sensitised cells, in a manner probably analogous to that of B lymphocytes described above. T lymphocytes can be divided into a number of subclasses with different properties; in the mouse these can be distinguished by the presence of a range of Ly antigens, a family of surface membrane markers. Some T cells, when sensitised, are capable of influencing the response of B cells to the relevant antigen.

These can be divided into 'helper' cells, which increase antibody response to antibody, and 'suppressor' cells, which decrease it. Under most common conditions of challenge with an exogenous antigen the net influence of T cells on B cells is stimulatory.

Suppressor T lymphocytes are important in the development of immune tolerance to an antigen, i.e. failure of antibody production following exposure to the antigen. This can occur with presentation of antigen via the gut; this aspect will be considered later (section 3). Still other sensitised T cells (cytotoxic T cells) will specifically kill cells which carry on their surface the antigens with which they react. T cells are recognisable in the laboratory by dividing in response to the mitogen phytohaemagglutinin (PHA), or by their ability to adhere to sheep red cells and form rosettes. Mature T and B cells continually circulate through the blood to the lymph nodes, spleen, and of particular interest here, to the Peyer's patches of the gut (described below). Those subsequently passing to afferent lymphatic vessels eventually rejoin the blood through the thoracic duct.

Antibodies

Antibody molecules, which are contained in the immunoglobulins, are one of the agents by which the immune system produces its effects. Their detailed structure need not concern us, only their functionally active parts. At one end of the molecule there is the antibody combining site, which, by virtue of a unique shape given to it by a specific amino acid sequence in its chain, has selective affinity for a particular antigen. At the other end, in the F_c fragment, there are regions which can combine with immune and phagocytic cells, or trigger the complement system. In man there are four main classes of immunoglobulin molecules, which are distinguished by structural differences in the main polypeptide chain; they are immunoglobulins G, A, M and E, usually written IgG, IgA, IgM and IgE.

The first three are, in order of decreasing concentration, the main classes in the serum. IgE, present in much less quantity, can have disproportionately large effects because of its ability to adhere to mast cells and sensitise them, causing 'immediate hypersensitivity' (Table 3.1). IgA is the immunoglobulin present in highest concentration in the gastro-intestinal and respiratory secretions. It is synthesised mainly by the plasma cells present in the gut wall, but also to some extent by those in lymph nodes and in the spleen. In man the circulating IgA is mostly a monomer, of 160,000 molecular weight, but secreted IgA is polymerised to a dimer by addition of an extra polypeptide, the J chain, synthesised in plasma cells. Secretory IgA also carries a further chain, the secretory component, which is synthesised by epithelial cells. This can join on to dimer IgA or to IgM and aid their transport across the epithelium, and has the important effect of rendering these molecules less susceptible to digestion. Small amounts of the other immunoglobulin classes are normally present in the intestinal secretions. There is no transport mechanism for them; however, inflammation of the gut can cause large quantities of IgG to leak into the gut lumen.

Table 3.1: Mechanisms of Immune Reactivity/Hypersensitivity

Type	Names	Mechanism	Examples
I	Anaphylactic Atopic	Antigen combining with IgE antibody fixed to a tissue mast cell, causing release of histamine and acute inflammation.	Pollen sensitivity (Hay fever) Dietary allergy
II	Cytotoxic	Antibody combining with a cell surface, aided by complement or phagocytic and similar cells.	Lysis and phagocytosis of bacteria. Lysis of red cells coated with anti-Rhesus antibody, in haemolytic disease of the newborn.
III	Arthus phenomenon Immune complex disease	Antigen antibody complexes in tissues either formed in situ or deposited from the circulation activate complement and generate inflammation.	Serum sickness following intravenous immunisation with a foreign protein.
IV	Delayed Cell mediated	Sensitised T lymphocytes react with an antigen causing cytotoxicity, lymphokine production or chronic inflammation.	Tuberculin reaction (sensitivity to tubercule bacillus product because of prior exposure). Nickel hypersensitivity.

When antibody molecules combine with antigens, aggregation of the antigen together with antibody follows because of the multivalent nature of the linkage. These aggregates are named immune complexes. All classes of antibody have this effect, which can lead to agglutination of particulate antigens, such as bacteria, or the formation of large precipitable aggregates of protein antigens. It is probably the aggregation together of the F_c portions of the antibody molecules that renders these portions biologically active, through the ability for multivalent binding with receptor molecules. Interaction of immune complexed antibody with phagocytic cells facilitates ingestion of the antigen into the cells and hence its final digestion. The *complement* system, which is a cascade of enzymes analogous to that for clotting, is activated by immune complexes, generating substances which provoke acute inflammation. If the antigen is part of a cell surface, for instance a bacterium, complement will fix to the surface and make the particle even more easily ingested by phagocytes and may even produce lysis of the bacterial cell. The activities possible vary with the immuno-globulin class of the antibody. Thus, IgG can adhere to phagocytic cells and fix complement; IgM will fix complement, and this can cause binding of the antigen to phagocytes, which is not possible with IgM antibody alone; IgA is only capable of activating complement when in high concentration and does not interact with phagocytes.

Effects of Immune Response

The ability of the immune system to damage cells and generate inflammation is necessary for its ability to destroy invaders. Occasionally the mechanisms involved lead to disease rather than protection from it, and it is perhaps ironic that they are described classically as 'hypersensitivity', taking the former point of view.

These mechanisms are summarised in Table 3.1 and illustrated in Figure 3.1. Type I reactions are produced by IgE antibody adhering to and sensitising tissue mast cells. Contact with antigen causes release of the mediator histamine from these cells, producing acute inflammation. If the response is generalised, anaphylactic shock follows; if localised, oedema and urticaria ('hives') result. This reaction does not have a definite role in body defence, though it may possibly contribute to immunity to parasites.

Antibody mediated lysis is the essential feature of the type II reaction. The cooperation of phagocytic or lymphoid cells, or of complement, is necessary, and this reaction is an essential means for the destruction of bacteria. It has been found recently that virus infected cells are also destroyed in this way, providing that antibody is present to viral antigens which appear on the cell surface.

Type III reactions are the result of the formation of antigen-antibody complexes. These are formed by the reaction together of multiple *antibody* molecules with multiple *antigenic* molecules. These may be large, insoluble ones formed in tissues, as in the Arthus phenomenon, when the activation of complement generates intense inflammation at the interaction site. Alternatively, circulating soluble

Figure 3.1: Diagrammatic Representation of the Four Types of Immune Reaction

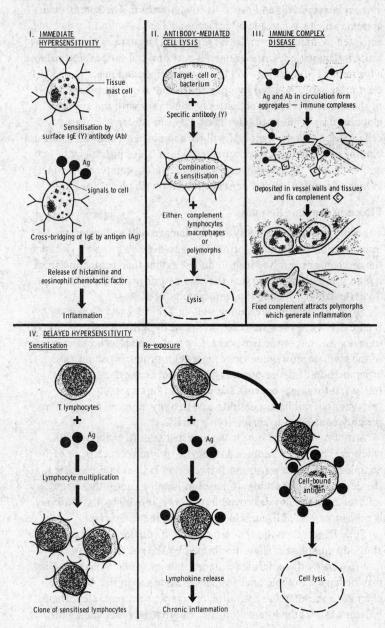

immune complexes may form in the blood, for instance in the serum sickness that follows the intravenous injection of a foreign protein. A more diffuse disease is produced; these complexes may also activate complement, and this generates inflammation wherever they deposit out of the circulation, for instance in the walls of arteries, in joints and in the skin. Glomerulonephritis (inflammatory kidney disease) is also produced, but for some unknown reason complement does not play any part in this. Complexes bearing complement are cleared rapidly by phagocytic cells, including the fixed phagocytes of the reticuloendothelial system in the liver, spleen, and bone marrow. Immune complexing of antigen aids its rapid removal from the blood-stream. Deposition of complexes with subsequent damage at sites outside the reticuloendothelial system can be regarded as an unwanted byproduct, due to overload of the normal clearance mechanism for the elimination of foreign antigen. Experimental methods for the detection of immune complexes in serum are now available.

Type IV reactions, delayed hypersensitivity, are the result of sensitised T cells meeting the antigen. Death of cells bearing the antigen and chronic inflammation are the consequences. Whether the reaction is beneficial or not depends on the nature of the antigen. If it is a pathogenic mycobacterium or a fungus, or a foreign graft, it will be eliminated. If it is the body's own protein altered by addition of a hapten (see below), such as nickel from a watch strap, a chronic eczematous hypersensitivity reaction will follow. Sensitisation of T cells to antigens can be tested experimentally by their uptake of tritiated thymidine during cell division provoked by exposure to the antigen (lymphocyte transformation), or by their production of lymphokines that affect other cells, as in the macrophage migration inhibition test.

Probably all these mechanisms play a part in immune diseases associated with the gut, and their relative contributions will be assessed in section 5.

3. The Immune System and the Gut

Lymphocytes and the Gut

The Peyer's patches of the gut are lymphoid aggregates in the submucosa and lamina propria of the intestine, with roughly similar structure and function to lymph nodes, with areas containing T and B lymphocytes (Figure 3.1). The lymphoid tissue of the appendix is similar. There are no afferent lymphatics to carry antigen to the immune cells, but instead there is a modification of the surface epithelial cells over the Peyer's patches. The surface of these cells consists of micro*folds*, rather than the micro*villi* which are normally found in epithelial cells, and they lack digestive, intracellular lysosomal enzymes. It seems that these modifications allow for easy access of gut antigens to the Peyer's patches, for soluble or even particulate antigens, such as Indian ink, pass freely into the upper 'dome' areas of the patches in rabbits.

The consequence of antigenic stimulation of these lymphoid cells differs from that in a lymph node. Peyer's patches lack the ability to form differentiated antibody-secreting plasma cells, a fact that may paradoxically render them susceptible to infection; the same may also be true of the appendix. B lymphocytes that are precursors of IgA plasma cells can, however, be found in them. These bear IgA molecules on their surface, but are not secretory.

The plasma cells of the lamina propria are derived from antigen stimulated lymphocytes of the Peyer's patches, but it is surprising that there is no efficient local route of migration from one to the other, and most of the cells travel by a most circuitous route. Gowans, in his Nobel prize winning discovery of the circulation of lymphocytes through the blood, lymph and thoracic duct, showed that the large lymphocytes of the thoracic duct home selectively to the lamina propria of the intestine, become plasma cells, and cease to circulate. In contrast the small lymphocytes continually recirculate, and are responsible for immunological memory. Most of the large cells are dividing lymphoblasts of the B lineage, and contain cytoplasmic IgA.

Where do these circulating cells bound for the gut originate? It is likely that the final answer is the Peyer's patches. Peyer's patch lymphocytes transferred from one rat to another can be found in the lamina propria six days after injection, where they become IgA secreting plasma cells. A problem arises over the timing of this migration. Large thoracic duct lymphocytes lodge in the gut within 20 hours, whilst few Peyer's patch cells are capable of arriving within this time. If mesenteric lymph node cells were tested in the same way, more can make a speedy journey. This suggests that Peyer's patch lymphocytes may rest and mature in the mesenteric nodes on their way to the thoracic duct; some also may travel on after a stop in the spleen. This indirect transfer of immune cells from Peyer's patches to the lamina propria has the advantage of spreading specific antibody secreting plasma cells from any challenged area to every part of the gut. They have even been detected in isolated loops of gut never in contact with antigen.

Figure 3.2: The Systemic Circulation and Maturation of Gut-derived Lymphocytes

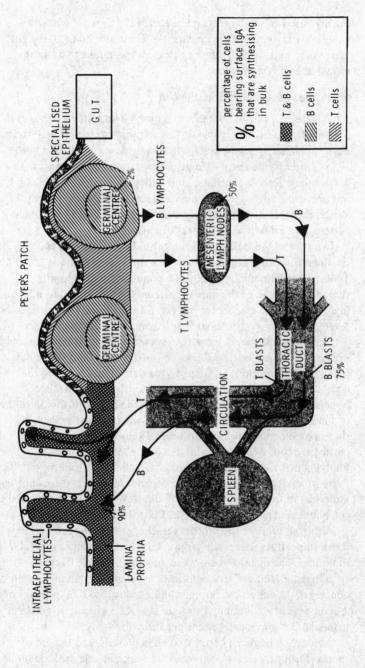

Finally, a few of the large lymphocytes of the thoracic duct are T lymphoblasts (lymphocyte precursors). These also home to the gut, where they migrate through the basement membrane to become intraepithelial lymphocytes.

Absorption of Antigens from the Gut

What is the role of this complex immune system of the gut? As even *particulate* material is capable of filtering through the gut wall to the Peyer's patches, it is now certain that the gut as a whole is at best a leaky barrier to the entry of large molecular weight substances. The gut contents act as a continual immunological challenge to the body, not only from pathogenic bacteria and viruses, but also from the antigenic proteins in the diet. Specialised mechanisms in the immune system have evolved so as to meet this attack.

Evidence of the leakiness of the gut to large molecules was first obtained from elegant immunological experiments in the 1920s and 1930s. Then immunology enjoyed a popularity, only recently surpassed, because of the hopes it offered for the control of infection in a pre-antibiotic era. Serum was taken from subjects suffering from severe allergy to foodstuffs such as fish and milk (see section on production of disease by immune responses). This contained cytophilic IgE antibodies and was capable of sensitising the skin of a normal individual on injection, by fixing to the dermal mast cells. In the classical Prausnitz-Kustner reaction, demonstrating immediate hypersensitivity, this sensitivity could be elicited by further injection of the antigen into the area, when acute inflammation ensued. In these experiments, however, the normal subjects *ate* some of the particular food. Acute inflammation in the test area followed, implying that the antigen had been absorbed intact from the gut. The route of absorption is variable, and depends in part on the size of the molecule. In the new-born calf, globulin (MW 160,000) is absorbed via the lymphatics, and insulin (MW 11,000) via the portal blood.

Although some of the protein absorbed may have been broken down to peptides that retain antigenicity, some remains as intact molecules. The quantities absorbed are only a minute fraction of the total ingested, but are very significant as far as the immune system is concerned. In one study, normal children absorbed 0.02 per cent of a 1 gram dose of ovalbumin. There are few other quantitative data in man, and this area clearly needs much further study.

Absorption has been better studied in animals, and the use of 'horse radish peroxidase' as the test substance has allowed the process to be followed by light and electron microscopy. About 0.01 per cent of a dose of peroxidase instilled into the jejunum of an adult rat was absorbed. This travelled through the intestinal epithelial cells by a pinocytotic process and the transport was reduced by metabolic inhibitors. This is the mechanism of entry under normal conditions, but any form of damage to the epithelium is likely to increase absorption by leakage between the cells.

Gut permeability is also increased in infancy, and in some animals, but not in man, there is a specific mechanism for the intestinal uptake of immunoglobulin from the colostrum.

Absorption even extends to particulate material, where it has been termed 'persorption'. Adult humans who managed to swallow 200 grams of raw oat flakes gained, for their pains, an average of 7 starch grains per ml of blood. Thus the body is exposed to a continual bombardment by a multiplicity of antigens from the gut, not only antigens from the diet, but also gut bacteria and their products.

Immune Responses and the Gut

The gut must have been quite a problem for the Almighty (or for evolution, depending upon one's philosophy), when the needs of the immune system were considered. Gut pathogens have to be effectively eliminated, and this ideally calls for an active immune response that can recruit potent inflammatory and destructive weapons. At the same time non-response to absorbed dietary antibodies might be theoretically preferable, to avoid the possible pitfalls of over-reactivity.

There are major differences in the immune response when stimulated via the gut rather than systemically. The first experimental observation was that the oral administration of a hapten produces a state of specific systemic tolerance. A hapten is a small chemical radical with which an antibody can specifically react, but is too small in itself to directly induce an immune response. It has to combine with a protein before it becomes active, and if administered uncombined may link with the proteins of the recipient. If picryl chloride or 2-4 dinitro chloro-benzene are injected into the skin, a cell mediated and antibody response normally follows, causing an inflammatory lesion at the site. Prior *ingestion* of the hapten prevents this sensitisation from taking place. This is known, after its discoverers, as the Chase-Sulzberger phenomenon. Recent work has shown that partial tolerance to soluble protein antigens can be produced similarly.

The liver has a central role in this phenomenon, as tolerance follows if the hapten is injected into the portal vein. If the portal and caval veins are transposed, thus bypassing the liver, no tolerance follows oral ingestion. The ability of Kupffer cells in the liver to take up aggregated material may be important, as aggregate *free* material tends to produce tolerance. Another factor may be the stimulation of an IgA class response from the intestinal plasma cells, as serum containing small quantities of these antibodies from orally immunised animals has induced tolerance to *parenteral* challenge following intraperitoneal injection. In animals neonatal exposure to dietary proteins is particularly effective in inducing long lived tolerance, but this does not apply in man.

The classical immune response on conventional parenteral immunisation (intramuscular, subcutaneous or intradermal) is much greater and longer on secondary and subsequent challenges with an antigen, compared to the primary response after initial exposure. Oral immunisation seems quite different. Experiments have been done in mice on the response by the immune cells of the spleen to orally ingested sheep red blood cells (SRBC). There was no increase in a secondary response over a primary; and neither was long lasting. More IgA antibody was produced after oral administration than after injection of the SRBC, possibly a relevant point in view of its 'tolerogenic' action mentioned above.

Despite these tolerance producing mechanisms, low levels of circulating antibodies to common dietary proteins are frequent in man. The majority of adults have antibodies to the proteins of cow's milk, to egg proteins, and to bovine and sheep proteins and cells. The levels of IgG antibodies are usually higher than IgA, but little IgM antibody is formed. Reaginic IgE antibodies to foodstuffs are occasionally formed in man, and can have dire consequences (see sections 2 and 6). Experimental animals are similar, except that the distribution of immunoglobulin classes of antibody produced varies both with the species and with the antigen used. It may well be that suppressor T cells are active in bringing about tolerance. Evidence that tolerance towards dietary antigens is an active state has been obtained in man; adults with low levels of dietary antibodies, despite a lifetime of exposure, produce poor antibody responses on parenteral immunisation with the same antigens. The gut immune system therefore avoids the Scylla of overreactivity by an innate tendency to induce systemic tolerance, so avoiding in particular the formation of IgG and IgM antibodies, which are potent in inducing inflammation and tissue damage. The local IgA antibody production has to steer the system away from the Charybdis of underreactivity by adequately coping with gastrointestinal infections.

The polyvalency of secreted IgA (and IgM) may allow for some discrimination between the reactivity with dietary antigens and pathogenic bacteria and viruses. The multiple linkages possible between a large particle with multiple antigenic sites, such as a bacterium, and a polyvalent antibody, enormously strengthens the *avidity* of the bond. With a small dietary protein antigen the possibilities for multiple bonding are much less, and the interaction and its consequences relatively diminished.

Oral immune challenge gives rise to a local secretory immune response within the gut as well as a systemic response. It is well known that gut infections, such as Shigella enteritis, give rise to detectable antibodies in the faeces before they appear in the serum. Immunity to gastrointestinal infection, e.g. poliomyelitis, is correlated with secreted rather than circulating antibody. Recent immunofluorescent studies have identified specific antibody-secreting plasma cells in the gut of animals after challenge, and determined their immunoglobulin class. These cells are derived from circulating immunoblasts (see above) and are mainly IgA secreting, as might be expected. Lesser numbers of IgM and IgG cells can also be found, and an occasional one secreting IgE. The antibodies are partly secreted into the gut lumen; the remainder pass to the gut lymphatics and portal blood.

A recent discovery is that much of the circulating IgA is excreted by the liver into the bile, and thence to the intestinal lumen. The half life of the IgA (6 days) in the blood is therefore very short compared to IgG (24 days), but the physiological advantage of secreting large quantities of IgA into the gut is obvious.

The efficiency of the secreted antibody in protecting the gut seems surprising, considering that it is mainly IgA which activates complement and phagocytic cells poorly. Bacterial lysis by IgA plus complement alone is not possible, but cooperation with the enzyme lyzozyme, to give lysis, has been reported. There is little doubt that the main actions are to clump bacteria, prevent their attachment to the intestinal wall and to combine with and so neutralise toxins.

Gut-derived Immune Complexes

Is the local response to dietary antigens of any use? Secreted antibodies in part remain trapped in the mucus layer lining the gut epithelium and will combine with antigen to form immune complexes. These complexes tend to remain in the mucus coat of the gut, and their presence there stimulates further mucus production. If the complexes are absorbed a greater proportion of the foreign protein is likely to be bound in the lamina propria than would occur in the absence of antibody. These effects together probably explain the decreased absorption of dietary proteins that has been observed in antibody producing animals. It therefore appears that the immune response does contribute to the exclusion of foreign material.

Any antigen that escapes into the circulation in the presence of an antibody response to it will be in the form of soluble immune complexes. These are avidly phagocytosed and eliminated by circulating and fixed phagocytes, especially if the aggregates are large. The Kupffer cells of the liver are well situated for the removal of complexes from the portal blood as it passes through the organ, and this must be an important duty of these cells.

It has even been suggested that the Kupffer cells of the liver and the antibody secreting cells of the spleen form a homoeostatic mechanism for elimination of gut derived antigens. Antigens from the gut will combine in the portal blood with antibodies from the spleen to form complexes; these will be removed by the Kupffer cells. Only if the antibody response is inadequate will antigen spill over into the systemic circulation, and thereby stimulate the spleen cells to make antibody. Clearly this cannot apply to antigen absorbed via the thoracic duct, thus by-passing the liver.

The immune complexing of antigen can be either a blessing or a curse. It aids the elimination of the antigen, but at the same time endows the antigen with potent pathogenic potential; if the complexes are not eliminated they may circulate in the blood, where they may produce disease at many sites, as in serum sickness (see section 2). In some circumstances, gut derived immune complexes can produce disease, and this will be considered in section 6.

4. Neonatal Nutrition and Development of the Immune Responses

Neonatal Immunity

A human infant is born with an immune system that is capable of responding to challenge. It is, however, inexperienced and therefore at first responds poorly. At birth, the levels of the serum immunoglobulins are low, except for IgG, which has been passively acquired from the mother by transfer across the placenta. This passive transfer of immunoglobulin containing antibodies is essential to tide the neonate over the critical first few months of life, before synthesis of immunoglobulin commences.

At birth IgM levels are 100 mg/L, one fifteenth of the normal adult value. Synthesis rapidly develops during the first months of life, and adult levels are almost attained by 6 months. IgG follows similarly by 12 months, but serum IgA is very slow, and development is not complete until adolescence (Figure 3.2). Evidence that lack of stimulation limits the development of the immune response in utero is given by the observed response to intrauterine infection. In such cases IgM levels can rise to equal those in adults. It seems that T lymphocyte responses in the neonate are well developed. These have been much more difficult to assess, but sensitisation in utero is probably unusual.

There is one gap in the innate immunological defences of the neonate — mucosal immunity. Passively transferred IgG is of little use as it is not actively secreted, and is liable to digestion. IgM levels are too low to be effective. Active secretory IgA immunity does develop rapidly, and specific IgA antibodies have been detected in the stool at 2 weeks of age, but clearly their induction must follow challenge, and there may be a critical gap.

The gut contents after birth are a most important source of antigen challenge, as they include potentially pathogenic bacteria and viruses, some, such as E. Coli, capable of causing fatal gastroenteritis. Once again, it is probably the lack of stimulation in utero that is responsible for the poor defences at birth. Congenital infection may induce IgA antibodies, and experiments in mice have shown that exposure to normal dietary and bacterial antigens is necessary for the normal development of mucosal immune cells, as cell numbers were much reduced in mice reared in germ free conditions.

Milk and Immunity

The importance of this subject to the nutritionist is in the appreciation of the role of human milk in supplementing this poor mucosal immunity of the neonate. The relative resistance to infection of children that are breast fed is now well established. There is a lower incidence of E. Coli gastroenteritis and encephalitis, of respiratory syncytial disease, and indeed of death from all causes (including sudden 'cot' death — see below).

There are multiple antibacterial and antiviral factors in human milk, of which IgA immunoglobulin is but one. Colostrum contains about 20 g/L of IgA, but the level falls with lactation to around 1 g/L. This

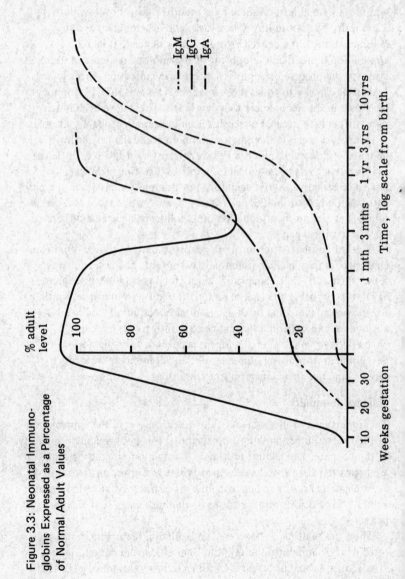

Figure 3.3: Neonatal Immunoglobins Expressed as a Percentage
of Normal Adult Values

IgA is synthesised by plasma cells of the mother's mammary gland. There is evidence that these cells may be derived from the circulating lymphoblasts derived from precursor gut lymphocytes. The feeding of nursing mothers with an avirulent strain of E. Coli rapidly caused IgA antibodies to that strain to appear in the milk. So this mechanism ensures that the baby has the benefit of its mother's experience — at least in immunological terms! Apart from the antibodies, there are also immunocompetent lymphocytes, phagocytic macrophages and complement components in milk which may be contributory.

The bacteriostatic effect of milk IgA antibody on E. Coli has recently been found to depend on synergy with another anti-bacterial factor, lactoferrin. This is an iron binding protein, with exceptional avidity for the metal, which deprives the bacteria of iron essential to their metabolism. Neither IgA nor lactoferrin alone are capable of inhibiting bacterial growth, but the combination is as effective as whole milk.

Lactoperoxidase is a non-specific factor capable of killing hydrogen peroxide producing bacteria, and may also be an important anti-bacterial agent. Antiviral, interferon-like activity, and other similar factors have been detected. The overall effect of breast milk is to replace potentially pathogenic gut flora such as E. Coli, clostridia and streptococci, by benign lactobacilli, but unfortunately this may be reversed on weaning.

There is no specific mechanism in man for the uptake by the gut of IgA from milk. This contrasts with ruminant animals, such as cows and sheep, where the entire transfer of immunoglobulins from mother to neonate is via the colostrum and gut uptake; the placenta is not permeable. Nevertheless, the human infant's gut is probably more 'leaky' to macromolecules than an adult's and this frequently leads to the formation of antibodies to absorbed dietary proteins, especially cow's milk proteins. Almost all children fed on cow's milk develop potent antibodies capable of precipitating in gel, a relatively insensitive laboratory test. The levels of milk antibodies decrease after the first year or two of life, but can persist at a low level in adults.

This immune response may include the formation of IgE antibodies and give rise to allergic conditions. Milk allergy with predominantly gastrointestinal symptoms is one, and will be discussed in full in section 6. This sensitisation has also been implicated in the cot death syndrome, as the frequency of IgE antibodies to the β-lactoglobulin of cow's milk, as well as to other non-dietary allergens, was found to be increased in the blood of infants dying of no apparent cause. Another abnormality of secretory immunity may also exist in this syndrome, as a marked decrease in secretory component has been reported at post mortem in the lungs of a group of children dying in this way. Respiratory syncytial virus infection was also found in some.

It might be asked whether the equivalent factors in cow's milk are not just as effective as those in human milk. However, bovine IgA antibodies are directed against bovine pathogens, not human, and are therefore largely irrelevant. Furthermore, pasteurisation and storage kill viable cells and lead to denaturation of anti-bacterial proteins.

The mechanisms leading to death in the 'cot death' syndrome remain controversial, and are probably multiple, but the nutritional message is clear — breast feeding reduces the risk. The benefits of breast feeding are twofold: it supplements the immune response and the avoidance of cow's milk prevents allergic sensitisation.

Neonatal Malnutrition

The general effects of malnutrition on the immune response will be considered in the next section, but there are particular effects in the neonatal period. The immunoglobulins in the fetus, as tested at birth in the cord blood, are abnormal. IgG is low compared to maternal blood, and IgM may be markedly increased. The latter is likely to be caused by intrauterine infection, brought about by lowered maternal resistance. Milk feeding usually continues for longer in underdeveloped countries where malnutrition is endemic, but the lessened volumes the mother produces result in poor transfer of passive immunity, even though the antibody level in the milk may be normal. Weaning is often followed by a period of repeated infections, because of the introduction of contaminated foods, the loss of passive immunity, and the alterations in gut flora. Malnutrition begins in utero and is expressed as growth retardation. It is not surprising that the mortality over the neonatal period correlates with the degree of retardation.

5. The Effect of Nutrition on the Immune Response

There is no doubt that malnutrition in man produces a severe defect in the function of the immune system. The consequent infections that develop are a burden that under-developed countries with poor standards of nutrition have to bear, and they hinder attempts to raise the standard of health. Furthermore, a vicious cycle develops: malnutrition depresses immunity, causing infection and infestation.

Infestation of the gut reduces food uptake, and chronic severe infections raise nutritional requirements by increasing nitrogen loss. In these ways infections increase malnutrition, and the cycle continues.

The extent of the problem can be seen from figures obtained by Suskind in Thailand. Ninety per cent of children with malnutrition had some form of infection. About half had pneumonia, and a third genitourinary tract infections. Most children had diarrhoea, but only in a quarter could pathogenic E. Coli or Shigella be cultured.

Measles is a severe disease in the malnourished child, the peak incidence being at 1 year, around the time of weaning. This disease accounts for 100,000 deaths a year in Nigerian children. These children are also riddled with parasites; in rural Nigeria 95 per cent have Ascaris, 30 per cent Strongyloides, 47 per cent Trichuris, 60 per cent Plasmodium falciparum and 12 per cent Entamoeba histolytica.

Malnutrition appears in the western world as a disease of the elderly and of certain hospital patients, in both of whom resistance to infection is lowered and an intact immune response is vital to wellbeing. One survey came to the alarming conclusion that half the surgical patients in a major American hospital were suffering from malnutrition, as measured by upper arm circumference and skinfold thickness. Depression of both T and B cell function was present in another group of hospital patients rendered malnourished by their illnesses, but normal immune function was restored by 18 days of intensive intravenous feeding.

The exact ways in which malnutrition affects the components of the immune response have been difficult to discover. In man the concurrence of malnutrition and infection confuses the issue, and ethics limit experimentation. However, a large number of sophisticated studies have thrown some light on the subject, enthusiasm, no doubt, fuelled by both the academic interest immunology generates and the immensity of the social problem. The subject has been extensively and excellently reviewed in a recent symposium,[1] *Malnutrition and the Immune Response*, edited by R. Suskind.

The syndromes of marasmus and kwashiorkor in children have been lumped together under the title 'protein calorie malnutrition'. Marasmus is characterised by severe wasting of muscle and adipose tissue, with good preservation of vital bodily functions, where any fall in serum albumin is slight. Kwashiorkor differs as there is oedema, sometimes of acute onset, hepatomegaly, desquamation of the skin, and frequent respiratory and alimentary infections. Serum albumin is severely decreased. The state probably represents one of decompensation of hepatic protein synthesis. Recent studies have suggested that essential fatty acid deficiency or jejunal bacterial colonisation, with villous atrophy, may be precipitating factors.

Experimental Malnutrition in Animals

The experimental evidence in animals strongly suggests that the immune system is damaged by lack of other dietary factors, such as folic acid and pyridoxine, as well as lack of protein and calories. Similar deficiencies also occur in man, for instance groups of Egyptian and South African children with kwashiorkor were also found to have pyridoxine deficiency. Therefore the range of dietary factors important in malnutrition has to be extended beyond only protein and calories, when the immune system is considered. The relative contributions of the various deficiencies towards immune malfunction and hence to disease in man are not known, and clearly must be determined.

The effect of malnutrition on the thymus has been known since the nineteenth century, when Simon, a physician, commented that the thymus was a 'barometer of nutrition and a very delicate one'. Gross atrophy and fibrosis of the thymus occurs in kwashiorkor; lymphoid tissue is also affected, with the thymus dependent areas depleted of cells. Similar but less severe changes are found in marasmus, and have been seen in experimental animals. The timing of the malnutrition is critical to the duration of the structural and functional defect. The growth of the thymus and spleen is partly by a programmed acquisition of new cells up to a certain age, for instance 65 days in the rat. Failure of this process through malnutrition results in a permanent cellular deficit. After this critical age the thymus cells are still very sensitive to malnutrition, but the defect can be reversed with refeeding. The extent to which the same is true for man is not certain, but it takes longer to reverse immunological defects which develop before rather than after one year of age.

The complexities of thymus lymphocyte function have made the results of animal experimentation hard to rationalise, and it must be remembered that the various T cell functions are performed by separate subpopulations of cells. Thus mice exposed for only two weeks at weaning to a reduced protein diet containing casein as 6 per cent of its total weight developed a permanent inability of their T lymphocytes, after sensitisation, to kill tumour cell targets. Similarly, severe atrophy of the thymus glands was produced in the litters of pregnant rats subjected to pyridoxine deficiency. Delayed hypersensitivity was tested in the skin of the offspring by sensitisation with dinitrochlorobenzene

(DNCB): the reaction was reduced, and the rejection time for skin allografts (i.e. grafts from genetically dissimilar members of the same species) was prolonged. Maternal deprivation of folic acid, B_{12}, choline and methionine (lipotrophic factors) had the same effect. Even a slight deficiency of these substances in utero resulted in diminished T cell responses, as seen by decreased PHA stimulation of the cells. Resistance to infection with Salmonella typhimurium was also diminished.

By contrast, workers at the Sloan Kettering Cancer Centre have conclusively shown that mice kept on a *moderate* restriction of protein develop *enhanced* T lymphocyte responses. An 8 per cent protein diet given to adult mice increases graft versus host reactivity, speeds allograft rejection, increases PHA induced lymphocyte transformation, and increased cytotoxic activity on tumour cells. Similar results were also obtained with rats and guinea pigs. Enhanced responses were only obtained with this moderate protein restriction. Severe deprivation, at 3 per cent of total diet, inhibited both T and B cell responsiveness.

Antibody responses in malnourished animals also show some ambivalence. With the chronic 8 per cent casein diet in mice, the response depended upon the nature of the antigen. Antibody production to brucella abortus was normal, but that to sheep red blood cells (SRBC) was depressed. The antibodies formed had lower affinity for antigen than those in normal animals. Total immunoglobulin in the blood was also decreased. Lipotrophic factor deficiency also decreased SRBC antibody production, despite the lack of any change in circulating B lymphocyte numbers. It is possible that a lack of co-operating helper T cells explains these results, as these are known to be required for SRBC antibody responses, but not for brucella antibody formation. This might suggest a differential effect of protein malnutrition on mouse T lymphocyte populations, as under similar conditions cytotoxic and graft rejection activities are increased. All the studies of protein deprivation on both T and B cells are complicated by the results obtained depending on the degree and duration of malnutrition. Acute, complete starvation actually *increases* antibody production.

Pyridoxine deficiency seems to produce a more severe overall damping effect on the immune system than protein malnutrition, for antibody production is decreased as profoundly as the thymus-dependent responses. This applies even to the antibody response to brucella, which is not thymus-dependent. Amino acid deficiencies usually depress antibody production more severely than T cell function, although both are affected.

Part of the enhancement of T lymphocyte cytotoxicity against tumour cells may be explained by an effect on antibody production. Inoculation of an animal with a tumour normally results in the formation of blocking antibodies, which partially prevent the ability of sensitised T cells to kill the tumour cells. The production of this antibody in mice was inhibited by a 3-11 per cent protein diet, and the intriguing result followed that these diets could inhibit the growth of experimental tumours.

To summarise, the evidence suggests that in experimental animals T lymphocyte responses are either enhanced or diminished by protein malnutrition, the actual effect depending on both the severity of the dietary restriction and the particular function studied. Cytotoxicity is most frequently enhanced and the activity of T cells cooperating with antibody most frequently diminished. Antibody responses are probably not primarily affected, unless the restriction is very severe, and failure of antibody production to some antigens may depend on the failure of co-operating T cells.

As might be expected from such a complex pattern of changes, there is no simple answer to the question of the effect of experimental malnutrition on susceptibility to infection. Liability to streptococcal and mycobacterial infections in mice was increased initially on 8 per cent casein, but largely returned to normal after 2-3 weeks. Influenza susceptibility showed a cyclical variation, and resistance to pseudorabies was increased. T cell immunity may be more important in combating viral rather than bacterial infections, but data and theory are unable to explain the situation fully at present.

Malnutrition in Man

In man the effects of malnutrition as seen in under-developed countries are most severe in the infant shortly after weaning. Breast feeding and late weaning protects the infant for the first year or so of life (see section 4). Despite the marked clinical and biochemical differences between marasmus and kwashiorkor which may then develop, the immunological differences are not great. There is a tendency for the functional deficits which develop to be more severe in kwashiorkor. For instance, BCG inoculation more frequently fails to induce tuberculin hypersensitivity. There is a much clearer distinction between a child who merely has malnutrition and one in whom the ill effects of malnutrition have been compounded by infection, a very common occurrence.

There is less contradiction to be found in the effects of malnutrition on T lymphocytes in humans than in animals. The majority of reports show a decrease in PHA induced transformation, in numbers of cells capable of rosetting spontaneously with sheep red cells and in delayed hypersensitivity. Some caution must, however, be observed in interpreting this observation at face value as evidence of depressed T cell function, for several factors interfering in these tests must be taken into account.

Skin tests for delayed hypersensitivity have shown depression of reactivity to a wide range of antigens in malnutrition. These include tuberculin, dinitrofluorobenzene (DNCB), and common bacterial, viral and fungal antigens. However, both viral and bacterial infections, and also associated endotoxaemia, can cause unresponsiveness in delayed hypersensitivity skin tests, even in normally nourished subjects. Thus the unreactivity in malnutrition might be due to concomitant infection, rather than the malnutrition itself. Inflammatory responses in the skin are depressed in malnutrition even to non-specific irritants (see below). In the absence of intact inflammatory mechanisms immune delayed hypersensitivity cannot be expressed; and the skin tests may be falsely negative. In addition to this failure of expression there is also a failure of initiation to sensitivity to new antigens.

Results with sheep cell tests are affected by the presence of C reactive protein, an acute phase glycoprotein in the serum of malnourished patients. The numbers of rosetting cells are decreased in malnutrition and the rosettes formed are smaller. More cells also remain which appear to have neither T nor B characteristics (null cells). The decreased numbers of rosetting cells would normally be taken to mean that the circulating T cells were decreased, but C reactive protein has been shown to decrease the ability of T cells to form rosettes. The null cells may be inhibited T cells. Other acute phase proteins which are immunosuppressive, such as alpha-acid glycoproteins, may also be involved. PHA transformation is not affected by C reactive protein, so may be a better indicator of T lymphocyte function. Despite these complicating factors, the weight of evidence suggests that T cell numbers and function are depressed in human malnutrition; thymic atrophy and depletion of thymus-dependent areas of lymph nodes are important structural features of this defect. Acute phase proteins and depressed inflammatory mechanisms may contribute to functional impairment of T lymphocyte activity.

B lymphocytes and antibody production are less affected by malnutrition. Numbers of B cells are largely unaltered and the levels of immunoglobulins of all classes show only moderate changes. Infection is the major factor affecting these levels; uninfected malnourished children may show a slight decrease, but in those with infection they are normal or elevated. IgE levels may be increased, particularly in those with parasitic infections. It is interesting that immunoglobulin protein synthesis is maintained even when that of other proteins, for instance albumin, is drastically reduced.

In contrast to the circulating immunoglobulins, there is a decrease in secreted IgA, necessary for defence against gastrointestinal and respiratory infections. IgA is decreased in nasal washings from a normal 24 per cent to about 16 per cent of total protein. The secretory antibody response to oral polio vaccines is approximately halved, and that to measles is also decreased. Antibody formation in malnutrition varies with the antigen tested. Normal antibody formation follows immunisation with tetanus and diphtheria toxoids, also after injection of pneumococcal polysaccharide or 'keyhole limpet haemocyanin', a favourite experimental immunogen. With yellow fever or killed influenza vaccines, or with experimental flagellin, tobacco mosaic virus or avian red cells, the responses were diminished. It is possible that the deficiencies in the latter group are due to lack of necessary T cell co-operation. In addition, infection has been found to have a marked immuno-suppressive effect on antibody formation, an effect that contributes to the vicious cycle of malnutrition and infection.

Complement, Polymorphs and Inflammation in Malnutrition

There are many other factors concerned in immunity to infection, apart from specifically immune lymphocytes and the antibodies they produce. Phagocytic cells and the complement system work in close cooperation with the specific mechanisms. Studies of the complement system in malnutrition have shown a loss of overall activity of the system, measured by its ability to lyse antibody coated red cells, and also that the levels of all but one of the individual components are decreased. Children with infections in addition to malnutrition have lower levels than those with uncomplicated malnutrition. There are probably two reasons for these changes. Between a quarter and a half of malnourished children have substances in their blood capable of combining with and activating complement. These are endotoxins and other factors derived from infecting bacteria. Nevertheless, complement levels are low in other children without these factors. In these it is likely that the heavy demands on protein synthesis made by the complement system cannot be met. Fortunately, all these abnormalities disappear rapidly with adequate food intake.

The importance of phagocytosis in defence lies in the removal and killing of micro-organisms. There are several stages to this process, firstly chemotaxic attraction of the phagocytic cells to their targets, then ingestion, and finally the intracellular stages of the handling of phagocytosed material. The first stage of chemotaxis is little affected in malnutrition; one 'skin window' study in kwashiorkor showed increased migration of polymorphs, but a decrease in monocytes; the total cell numbers were slightly increased. In vitro tests have shown some mild defects. The next stage, ingestion, and the intracellular vacuole formation that follows are normal. The final event in the chain, bacterial killing, may be defective. Reports on this stage have varied greatly and the decisive factor is most probably the presence or absence of infection. This was shown clearly in a study on Indian children, where malnutrition plus infection grossly inhibited bacterial killing by polymorphs. The defect was much greater than with either alone, and reached the very low levels seen in the rare congenital 'chronic granulomatous disease'.

Extensive biochemical investigations have been made in the search for polymorph abnormalities in malnutrition. The levels of most enzymes involved have proved to be normal, with the exception of the activity of the hydrogen peroxide/myeloperoxidase/halide bacterial killing system, which is decreased. This is significant, as in general it correlates well with bactericidal ability. High resting levels of hexose monophosphate shunt metabolism and of nitro-blue tetrazolium reduction suggest that pre-existing in vivo phagocytosis and infection are affecting the cells.

Many aspects of the body's design contribute non-specifically to resistance to infection. The normal microbial flora, the body secretions and the barriers of skin and mucosa provide passive resistance to the establishment of pathogens. If infection arises, then inflammatory, endocrine, metabolic and febrile responses aid in combating it. Several of these are damaged in malnutrition. Vitamin A, those of the B complex, and Vitamin C, as well as protein and zinc, are required to maintain the integrity of skin and mucosa. The lack of these substances in malnutrition is responsible for the desquamation and ulceration of the skin frequently seen, which allows the entry of micro-organisms. Colonisation of the stomach and small bowel with anaerobic organisms occurs and is associated with malabsorption and diarrhoea.

The inflammatory response is greatly suppressed in malnutrition. Edelman and colleagues found this accidentally when attempting to assess delayed hypersensitivity in malnutrition by skin tests with dinitrofluorobenzene (DNFB). This compound in 2 mg doses has a direct non-immunological irritant action on the skin, normally causing an acute inflammatory reaction after 2 days. Only 13 out of 30 children with marasmus and kwashiorkor were able to give this response. Further evidence of lack of inflammatory response was obtained from the failure of passive sensitisation of severely malnourished children by allergic serum (see section 2). Improved nutrition produces a rapid return of the inflammatory response to normal.

In acute infection there is normally an increase in the synthesis of acute phase glycoproteins by the liver, probably induced by a leucocyte derived mediator. The best known of these is C reactive protein, named after its affinity for pneumococcal C polysaccharide. Virtually all children with kwashiorkor show increased levels of this protein, which return rapidly to normal with an improved diet. It seems unlikely that the increased levels and their rapid return to normal are explained entirely by pre-existing infection, but no alternative mechanism is known. The functions of these proteins are not fully understood, but may include an immunosuppressant effect, as they are known to react with and inhibit T lymphocytes (see above).

The importance of the inflammatory deficit in malnutrition cannot be overestimated, and is probably the final common pathway of predisposition to infection. The integrity of the immune, phagocytic and complement systems is necessary for a normal inflammatory response to a micro-organism. The phagocytic and complement systems are necessary even for a stimulus, such as an inert foreign body, that does not induce specific immunity. The defects in these systems, and the immune system, probably explain the inflammatory deficit in malnutrition, but more information is necessary. Recent work has suggested that zinc deficiency may be important. Infection itself may have an immunosuppressant or anti-inflammatory effect (see above), and high plasma cortisol levels in kwashiorkor might be contributory.

Response to Infection

The response to infection in malnutrition is abnormal. Frequently there is tissue necrosis and widespread dissemination of pus-forming organisms, with minimal tissue reaction; normally a localised purulent lesion would be produced. The processes of healing and repair are depressed, for instance tropical sores in the malnourished do not heal until the diet is improved. The tissue response in malnutrition has been compared to that in immunodeficiency states, for instance in the atypical response to measles, with giant cell formation and pneumonia.

Children with kwashiorkor are frequently apyrexial or even hypo-thermic when infected. This can be explained by the lack of formation of pyrogen from the child's polymorphs through depressed metabolism and a poor inflammatory response. Infections in these circumstances are frequently fatal. The failure of these normal responses leads to the increased susceptibility of malnourished subjects to infection, but the close association of malnutrition with infection itself has made for practical difficulties in attributing an exact cause to the abnormalities found.

Vaccination

The extent to which the painstaking studies described above will improve the treatment of malnutrition is an open question, but already the development of suitable national vaccination programmes for countries with endemic malnutrition has been one practical consequence of the study of immunity in malnutrition. Responses to cholera, yellow fever, and influenza vaccines are depressed in malnutrition, so probably there is little to be gained from their use. Poor immune responses cause the infections with living vaccines to be more severe than normal, and in infants up to 6 months vaccines cause a significant strain on nutritional status, which may precipitate weight loss. For practical reasons any vaccination programme must be simple. The Pan American Health Organisation in 1969 recommended a two-visit vaccination schedule (1) diphtheria, tetanus and pertussis triple vaccine (DTP), oral polio and BCG. (2) DTP, oral polio, smallpox and measles, to be carried out in the first two years of life.

Overnutrition and Lipids

To take the other side of the coin, a reduced resistance to infection has also been identified in overnutrition. Rats succumb more easily to malaria and tuberculosis, and chickens to pneumococcal infections when taking a high fat diet. Obese children also appear more liable to chest infections. Not a great deal is known about detailed immune mechanisms in over-nutrition. One study with overfed monkeys showed a defect in phagocytosis. This can be correlated with other studies which have shown that ingested ethyl stearate and glycerol trioleate hinder the clearance of carbon particles from the blood by the reticuloendothelial system. It may be that excess chylomicrons (fat particles) in the blood are phagocytosed, and divert the attention of the macrophages from other particles, including bacteria. Perhaps this is the rationale of the old adage 'feed a cold and starve a fever'.

The effects of lipids on the immune response extend even further. Methyl palmitate and cholesterol oleate given orally diminish antibody responses to sheep red cells; this might again be via inhibition of macrophage function. A particular immunosuppressive role has been claimed for polyunsaturated fatty acids. Linoleic acid is capable of prolonging the survival of skin allografts in mice; it reduces the cytotoxic responses of splenic lymphocytes and depresses lymphocyte transformation with PHA — all T lymphocyte functions. These observations may be relevant to the use of polyunsaturated fat enriched diets for the treatment of arterial disease in man. One study showed an apparent increase in malignant tumours in men so treated, and it was postulated that immune surveillance and destruction of tumour cells had been inhibited. However, subsequent reports have not confirmed that this danger exists. There may be some advantage in the use of linoleic acid as an immunosuppressant after renal transplantation.

6. Production of Disease by Immune Responses Related to the Diet and the Gut

The normal secretory and systemic immune responses to dietary and other gut content antigens have been described in section 3, and the mechanisms by which immune responses can produce disease in section 2.

Circulating Antibodies

The levels of circulating antibodies to dietary proteins of the major immunoglobulin classes have been intensively studied in many diseases, especially those that are diet and gut related. The methods used in the past have not been entirely satisfactory. The only highly sensitive method used, haemagglutination, suffers from non-specificities that have led to positive results, for instance in ulcerative colitis, which have not been confirmed subsequently. Quantification of the antibody levels in absolute terms is difficult and has not been attempted to any extent with dietary antibodies. Increased antibody levels are found in coeliac disease, milk allergy, aphthous ulceration, gastric atrophy, cystic fibrosis, malnutrition, selective IgA deficiency and liver disease. The detection of IgE class antibodies is a separate issue, and will be considered later in connection with food allergy.

Although there are high titres of gluten antibodies in gluten sensitive enteropathy (coeliac disease) and of milk antibodies in milk allergy, individual antibodies are not specific to particular diseases. Gluten antibodies for instance are also found in ulcerative colitis, admittedly usually less frequently and in lower titres. In any one disease multiple antibodies can usually be demonstrated to a range of antigens. Antibodies are commonly found to the major proteins of the diet, such as the lactoglobulin and lactalbumin of cow's milk, bovine serum albumin, and ovalbumin. Therefore dietary antibodies are not a specific marker for any disease, and so are of little diagnostic significance.

There are two possible explanations of this widespread increase in dietary antibodies in certain diseases. Firstly, abnormal permeability of the gut epithelium in gut disease, because of inflammation and ulceration, may lead to increased entry of dietary antigens and hence to a greater challenge to and response of the immune system. Increased dietary antibodies are also found in gastric atrophy and cystic fibrosis, where more undigested protein reaches the intestine. Likewise in liver disease high levels of dietary and bacterial antibodies are found, probably because of impaired phagocytosis and breakdown of dietary antigens in the liver. Failure of the destruction of mitogenic endotoxins derived from gut bacteria may also play a part by allowing their direct stimulatory action on antibody producing cells. The accidental inhalation of milk proteins in children was found to be associated with the formation of precipitating antibodies. Antigens are well absorbed from the lungs, and this again supports the hypothesis.

The second possible explanation is that the dietary antibodies are a coincidental marker of an overreactive immune system. This could be producing disease by quite separate mechanisms, for instance by autoimmunity against the body's own components. The primary cause could be a defect in immune regulation, for instance in suppressor T lymphocyte function.

It has been suggested that the local immune response in an inflamed gut could produce significant circulating antibody. As IgA antibodies are made in the gut, while mostly IgG dietary antibodies appear in the circulation, it seems an improbable explanation.

Immune Complexes

Dietary antibodies may combine with absorbed antigens to form immune complexes (see sections 2 and 3). Circulating immune complexes have been detected in the serum in 33-100 per cent of patients with coeliac disease, in 30-80 per cent with dermatitis herpetiformis, in 50 per cent with ulcerative colitis and in 28-35 per cent with Crohn's disease, all diseases with abnormalities of the small intestine or colon. The frequency has varied with the methods employed and probably depends mainly on their relative sensitivities. Recent work has shown complexes to be present in all patients with coeliac disease and dermatitis herpetiformis, when the results of several methods were combined.

Unfortunately, techniques have not yet advanced far enough to allow for the detection of the antigen involved in the complexes, except in special cases. One might predict that the complexes formed in gut disease consist in part of dietary or bacterial antigens absorbed from the lumen, together with the corresponding antibody. There is good evidence for this in one condition, arthritis complicating a surgically induced ileal bypass, performed to treat intractable obesity. Circulating immune complexes were discovered and were unusual in separating from the serum on cooling, i.e. were 'cryoglobulins'. The separated cryoglobulins contained much higher concentrations of antibodies to gut bacterial antigens than the whole serum, suggesting that the antigens themselves were also present. It is not known, however, why ileal shunting should lead to immune complex formation.

Circulating soluble immune complexes are a heterogeneous category of circulating aggregates of varying size, containing antibodies of any class, with or without the ability to activate complement. Variations in these characteristics can cause complexes to range from the totally innocuous to those which are dramatically pathogenic, for example in acute post-streptococcal kidney disease. The principal mechanism in many diseases is the activation of complement with the subsequent generation of inflammation.

It is in the peripheral complications of gut diseases that immune complexes are most likely to play a significant role. Ulcerative colitis and Crohn's disease can be complicated by arthritis, skin lesions, liver damage and inflammation of the eye, which are probably all immune complex mediated. Immune complexes of gluten complexed with anti-gluten antibody have been demonstrated in the skin lesions of dermatitis herpetiformis, which may be associated with coeliac disease, another instance where the antigen in the complex is known (see below). There is the possibility that insoluble immune complexes may be formed in the gut from antibodies to gluten and ingested gluten, and the consequent Arthus phenomenon may contribute to the lesions of coeliac disease (see below). A similar mechanism has also been proposed in ulcerative colitis, where increased levels of antibodies to anaerobic bacteria are present, together with autoantibodies to colonic tissue.

Dietary Antibodies and Atheroma

A controversial issue was raised by Davies and others, who found that antibodies to milk and egg proteins, as tested by tanned cell haemagglutination, were increased in patients with myocardial infarction. He suggested that atherosclerosis and thrombosis might be produced by an immune mechanism, possibly the formation of immune complexes from absorbed dietary antigens. Some subsequent studies using haemagglutination confirmed the observations, others did not, and radioimmunoassay results were negative. The explanation of these discrepancies is not apparent, but may possibly arise from non specificities of the haemagglutination technique.

Recently, however, Taylor and Muir studied experimental atherosclerosis in rabbits fed a high lipid diet plus one of two preparations of soya bean meal, having low and high antigenicity. Their initial report on the study showed that there was a good correlation between the antibody response to soya bean meal and the degree of atherosclerosis induced. Circulating immune complexes were detected and were positively correlated with the antibody levels. The animals with the highest titres developed giant cell arteritis, a pathology not previously produced by an experimental method. The antibody response to soya bean meal appeared unusually large for a dietary antigen, and might have been enhanced by the absorption of mitogenic lectins in the beans causing direct stimulation of antibody forming cells. Further development of this work should be interesting.

Food Allergy

Abnormal reactions to foodstuffs are known as food *intolerance,* and this includes non immune disease mechanisms, such as the deficiency of the intestinal enzyme lactase, producing one form of milk intolerance. The term food *allergy* is reserved for conditions where a specific immune reaction is thought to occur. By convention this can be divided into gastrointestinal allergy, when reactions occur in the gut, and somewhat paradoxically, alimentary allergy, when symptoms such as urticaria and angio-oedema are seen at distant sites.

An acute anaphylactic attack is the most severe and dramatic, but fortunately rare, form of allergic response. This occurs at the time of ingestion of the allergen, or shortly afterwards. Potentially fatal acute angio-oedema, difficulty in breathing, cyanosis and a fall in blood pressure are produced, sometimes with chest pain and electro-cardiographic abnormalities. Alternatively vomiting, abdominal pain and diarrhoea can be the main symptoms. A skin rash is nearly always present, and may be the dominant symptom in less severe attacks.

Apart from these rare acute cases, the disease is of greatest severity in young children. Cow's milk is the principal allergen and the symptoms produced, in order of frequency are — diarrhoea, vomiting, nasal obstruction, atopic dermatitis, abdominal pain, asthma, urticaria and anaphylaxis. Malabsorption or a protein losing enteropathy may be produced, and failure to thrive is an important consequence. There may be subtotal or complete villous atrophy of the small gut; sometimes there is eosinophilia of the blood and of the lamina propria. Although it is important to distinguish this condition from milk intolerance through lactase deficiency, sometimes a secondary lactase deficiency can arise as a *consequence* of the villous atrophy. In adults with allergy, distant symptoms usually predominate, although occasionally malabsorption or protein losing enteropathy occur. It is interesting that there have been several reports of asthma being attributed to food allergy, although estimates of the frequency of this cause have varied widely.

Table 3.2: Examples of Foodstuffs Causing Allergy*

Meats	beef, lamb, pork, chicken
Fish	halibut, tuna fish, smelt, salmon, perch, lobster, shrimp, oysters, clams, cod liver oil
Vegetables	carrot, pea, potato (raw), soya bean, spinach, runner bean, cabbage, broccoli, mustard, onion, asparagus, cauliflower, ginger
Fruits	apple, apricot, banana, orange, peach, pear, pineapple, prune, tomato, strawberry
Cereals	barley, maize, oats, rice, rye, wheat
Nuts	peanuts, walnut
Misc.	coffee (green), castor seed, milk — cow and goat, eggs
Food additives	penicillin, tartarazine dye, limonene oil, benzoic acid

*Note: The immunological nature of the intolerance has not been definitely established in all cases.

A very wide range of food substances has been found to induce allergy (Table 3.2), but the overall incidence of this type of allergy is low compared to others: about 0.5 per cent of the population — and maximal in childhood. Bleumink experimented extensively on the nature of the active substances in food allergens and fully reviewed the topic in 1970. Some of the allergens show similarities, with molecular weights in the range 17,000-40,000; several are spontaneous chemical condensation products formed between lysine residues on proteins and carbohydrates (Table 3.3). These have characteristic ultraviolet absorption spectra, and show blue fluorescence. This condensation reaction occurs on storage and is known as non-enzymic browning, or the Maillard reaction.

Table 3.3: Identification of Allergenic Substances

Food	Allergen	Notes
Cow's milk	β Lactoglobulin	Maillard condensation products have increased activity (Bleumink).
Hen's eggs (white of)	Ovomucoid and other proteins	Trypsin inhibitor, heat stable.
Shellfish	Sarcoplasmic protein M	Heat stable.
Tomato (ripe)	Polydisperse glycoproteins	Maillard condensation products.

Knowledge that the mechanism of food allergy is immunological dates back to the classical studies of Prausnitz and Kustner in 1921. In the original study Kustner was allergic to cooked fish, and his serum would on injection confer sensitivity on Prausnitz's skin, which could be tested by the injection of fish extract into the same area. This led to the recognition of tissue fixing 'reaginic' antibodies, now known to be IgE, as mediators of this reaction (see section 2). Likewise by injecting serum from a patient sensitive to peanuts, it proved possible to sensitise the gut at a colostomy site.[2] The recipient then *ate* peanuts and within minutes acute inflammation developed simultaneously at both the colostomy and similarly sensitised skin sites. This shows that a Type I hypersensitivity reaction can occur in the gut. As the inflammation developed before the peanuts themselves had passed the stomach, the allergen must have reached the colostomy through the blood stream, a remarkable demonstration of the facility of absorption of undigested antigens!

Skin testing by a prick test with the allergen has been the standard means of diagnosing food allergy for many years, but has not always proved satisfactory. A high percentage of normal subjects can give positive reactions, for instance 75 per cent to casein and 16 per cent to milk protein in one study.

In a recent survey, Chua and others found that in food allergy the

prick test correlated with the history in 76 per cent, the passive
sensitisation of guinea pig lung by serum in 37 per cent, and radio-
immunoassay on serum detecting IgE antibody to the allergen in 54 per
cent. Because of the tissue fixing ability of IgE antibodies the serum
levels are extremely low, and even the great sensitivity of radio-
immunoassay is only just sufficient for their detection; perhaps low
levels are missed, even by this technique.

Although IgE mediated Type I hypersensitivity is the most important
mechanism in food allergy, other immune mechanisms may play a
significant part in some cases. Delayed hypersensitivity (Type IV) to
para aminobenzoic acid, acquired through use of suntan lotion, may
produce eczema. Ingestion of foodstuffs containing benzoic acid used
as a preservative, or related compounds, can cause an exacerbation of
the eczema. Type III reactions may occur in milk allergy, as high levels
of milk antibodies are present, and complement activation in the
serum has been observed following milk challenge. This suggests that
antibody-antigen combination has taken place, and raises the
possibility that damage to the gut may be produced by an Arthus
phenomenon. The numbers of IgA and IgM secreting cells in the lamina
propria of the gut are over twice the normal in this condition. Peripheral
disease may also be caused by this mechanism, for Heiner in 1960
recognised a rare association between high milk antibodies and
pulmonary disease. In milk allergy, positive lymphocyte transformation
with milk proteins suggests that even cell mediated immunity could be
involved.

In adults, avoidance of the sensitising food is the only useful treatment. Fortunately, children usually grow out of milk allergy, but
treatment with replacement diets can be complicated by the child
developing allergies to them, for instance to soya bean protein.

Many hypotheses have been made concerning the aetiology of
dietary hypersensitivity. Early exposure to antigenic diets by bottle
feeding has been implicated, through finding an increased risk compared
to breast feeding. IgE antibody matures early in development and
adult levels are seen in the blood soon after birth. Therefore, antigenic
exposure before immunoglobulin synthesis of other classes has
matured might cause the antibody response to be more of this class.
Further support for this notion is that transient IgA deficiency at 3
months of age was found to be associated with the later development of
atopy. This deficiency might also cause increased absorption of antigen,
through failure of exclusion by secretory antibody, and hence a greater
stimulus to IgE production. The onset of allergy has been seen after

attacks of infectious gastro-enteritis in infants, and again greater absorption through the inflamed gut could be involved.

Soothill has suggested that other defects of the immune response lead to greater stimulation of IgE production by failing to eliminate antigen effectively. Such abnormalities as low affinity antibody, poor macrophage function and complement defects have this effect. It is interesting in this context that as long ago as 1923 an excellent study showed cow's milk allergy in 80 out of 98 children with marasmus. The multitudinous defects of the immune response in malnutrition, including low affinity antibody, complement deficiency, and defective phagocytosis were described in section 4. Nevertheless, other factors such as parasitism and damage to the gut could provide alternative explanations. There is also an apparently inherent disorder of the blood basophils in food allergy. They have been found recently to have a high spontaneous release of histamine, and it is therefore possible that this inherent instability of the cells may magnify the effect of otherwise trivial sensitivity.

There is an impressive body of evidence that IgE antibody production is under the control of suppressor and helper T cells, and in contrast to Soothill's view, E. Jarrett has found that very low doses of antigen are required in animals to obtain IgE responses. In greater doses tolerance is produced, probably through the action of specific suppressor T cells. She postulated that a relative deficiency in this regulation is the prime defect in atopy, and that the peak incidence of food allergy seen in children under 4 years is due to a belated maturation of this cell population.

Clearly, further information is needed before the question of the mechanism responsible for dietary allergy can be answered, particularly on the absorption of dietary proteins in normal and allergic subjects. The detection and quantification of food antigens in serum by radio-immunoassay might be rewarding.

The Role of Dietary Allergy in Other Diseases

There is a long standing controversy over the role of milk allergy in ulcerative colitis. The disease is probably associated with other allergies, and a controlled trial has shown clinical improvement on a milk free diet. The drug sodium dicromoglycate, which inhibits immediate hypersensitivity, is also of benefit. On the other hand, no serum IgE antibodies to milk have been detected and Buisseret and others have recently found an acute, possibly non-immunological, intolerance to milk and other foods in some colitic patients, which

causes diarrhoea and vomiting. Circulating prostaglandin levels increased
on challenge, and the condition responded dramatically to aspirin
treatment. Similar findings were also made in some patients with gastrointestinal allergy. Still another possibility in the aetiology of ulcerative
colitis is that of a transmissible agent. The position is uncertain, and no
definite role for allergy has been established.

Steroid sensitive nephritis that shows 'minimal change' of glomeruli
on renal biopsy is associated with a state of atopy, including milk
allergy. Serum antibodies to milk proteins may also be increased. In a
recent study challenge with milk after a period of withdrawal caused
an exacerbation of the disease. Immune complexes have also been
found in the serum, but do not localise in the glomeruli or fix
complement, unlike those causing other forms of nephritis. Nothing is
yet known of their antigenic components, or of their possible
pathogenic role in this disease.

Coeliac Disease

Gluten intolerance, as manifest in coeliac disease of children and
adults, is characterised by a villous atrophy of the jejunum associated
with malabsorption that is reversible on the withdrawal of gluten from
the diet. It is the gliadin fraction of gluten that is toxic; this is the
wheat protein that is soluble in 70 per cent aqueous ethanol, and
which in turn consists of several distinct proteins that can be separated
by electrophoresis or ion exchange chromatography. Only the alpha
gliadin is toxic, and activity is also present in Frazer's fraction III,
which is a pepsin and trypsin digest of gluten. The gluten of rye, barley
and oats can also damage the gut.

There has been a long standing controversy over the aetiology of
the disease, the rival theories being an enzyme defect or an immune
mechanism; abnormal affinity of gluten for cells may also enter the
picture. In recent years Falchuk and colleagues have carried out an
ingenious series of experiments that throw light on this enigma. Jejunal
biopsies were cultured and the initial and final levels of alkaline
phosphatase enzyme, derived from epithelial cells, measured. In
normal specimens there was an increase during culture and the same
took place in active coeliac specimens, only with a lower initial value.
If a peptic tryptic digest of gliadin were added to the culture medium,
the enzyme increase was inhibited in the active coeliac, but not in the
control. This was attributed to epithelial cell damage by the digest.
If, however, a specimen was taken from a symptom-free coeliac
patient in remission on a gluten free diet, the enzyme levels behaved

normally in the presence of gliadin. This implies that the defect producing the disease is not an *intrinsic* disorder of the coeliac mucosa, but only arises on protracted exposure to gluten in vivo, when a response occurs.

In further experiments two biopsies were cultured together, so as to test for the presence of soluble mediators. If an active coeliac was put with an inactive, then the enzymes of the inactive patient were inhibited in the presence of gluten, whereas an active coeliac had no effect on a normal control. Therefore, a soluble mediator must have been present, but could only act on a potential coaeliac mucosa. Taking these results at face value, and putting them together, it seems that two factors are necessary to produce mucosal damage. Firstly, a slow response to gluten that takes place in vivo; this might well be immunological. Secondly, a difference, possibly genetic, has to exist in the mucosa. On the other hand, recent studies on inherent enzymic abnormalities in the mucosa have been negative.

There are many immunological abnormalities in coeliac disease. The lamina propria of the gut contains an increased cell population, part of a local inflammatory reaction. There are large numbers of plasma cells, followed in number by lymphocytes, macrophages, eosinophils and mast cells. Intraepithelial lymphocytes are also increased. The total number of immunoglobulin containing cells (plasma cells) in a standard length of mucosa increases 2.5 times, IgG producing cells increase from 2.6 to 8 per cent, IgM from 17 to 20 per cent, and IgA drops from 81 to 72 per cent. A rare but interesting exception to this is that 1 in 50 coeliac patients have *total* IgA deficiency, a frequency many times that in the normal population. There is increased immunoglobulin synthesis, and this amounts to a two to five fold increase on gluten challenge in a treated patient. A large part of this increase is actually anti-gluten antibody.

Complement components and IgA can be seen in the lamina propria on gluten challenge, suggesting that an antibody-antigen reaction has taken place, and that the mucosal damage could be produced by an Arthus type reaction (Type III hypersensitivity). Findings in the circulation parallel those in the mucosa; there are high levels of antibodies to gluten, but their lack of specificity to coeliac disease was noted above. Consumption of circulating complement is produced on challenge with gluten, and circulating immune complexes have been demonstrated by several different tests. This supports the hypothesis that an antigen-antibody reaction takes place on challenge, mainly in the gut mucosa, but with some spill-over into the circulation.

'Dermatitis herpetiformis' is associated with gluten sensitive enteropathy, and is probably produced by immune mechanisms. About three quarters of those with this skin disease have gut mucosal changes, often mild and without clinical effect. The skin lesions consist of urticarial subepidermal bullae, with an eosinophil and neutrophil infiltrate, and they regress slowly on a gluten-free diet. Immuno-fluorescence shows IgA and other antibodies fixed in the dermal papillae, with more being found, curiously, in non-affected than affected skin. The C3 component of complement is, however, more often present in the lesions than elsewhere.

Both in coeliac disease and dermatitis herpetiformis circulating antibodies are present that react with connective tissue reticulin. There is at least partial cross reactivity between reticulin and gluten, so the reactivity may be due to gluten antibodies. Reticulin is however also present in meat of the diet and the antibody could arise from this source of stimulation.

Circulating immune complexes that are complement fixing have been found in 80 per cent of untreated patients with dermatitis herpetiformis, but in only 36 per cent of those on a gluten-free diet. Local factors, for instance inflammation or special affinity for the structure, are important in directing immune complex tissue damage to a particular site. Gluten containing immune complexes may therefore be predisposed to fix in the skin because of affinity of the antibody in the complex for dermal reticulin. Activation of complement will then generate local tissue damage. More simply, circulating antireticulin or antigluten antibodies might have the same effects by direct combination, although autoantibodies by themselves rarely seem capable of much tissue damage. In some other autoimmune diseases, such as thyroid disease, cell mediated immunity has proved more important, but this has not so far been assessed in dermatitis herpetiformis.

In coeliac disease, early attempts to find T lymphocyte sensitisation to gluten were unsuccessful, but recently Sikora and others found that a highly refined subfraction of Frazer's fraction III would stimulate lymphocytes to divide. Subsequently Douwes showed sensitisation of leucocytes by the production of a migration inhibition factor on exposure to gluten in an agarose medium. This reaction clearly distinguished coeliac patients from normals.

The question remains, why do only certain people develop coeliac disease whilst the vast majority are unaffected? There is a known genetic predisposition to the disease, and advances in the study of the HLA (human leucocyte antigen) system have been very revealing. This is a genetic system consisting of four loci with multiple alleles at each, controlled by genes on chromosome six. The alleles are expressed as surface markers on leucocytes, which can be recognised serologically. The HLA-B8 antigen is found in about 20 per cent of normal Caucasians. In coeliac disease, there is a very significant increase to 70 per cent of those affected. Though this relationship is clearly of great interest, one has to remember that the vast majority of people with B8 will not get coeliac disease.

More recently a much stronger association has been found with a newly discovered variety of HLA antigen that is found only on B lymphocytes. Antisera recognising this antigen, named DRW3, react with the cells of about 80 per cent of patients with coeliac disease, but with no normal controls. These D series antigens are associated with genes controlling the immune response, so this evidence supports the view that an abnormal immune response is associated with this disease. One possibility is that the immune response could be modified because the antigen on the B lymphocyte is a receptor for gluten binding. No direct support for this idea exists, but it is interesting that there is evidence that the epithelial cells of the intestine specifically bind gluten in coeliac disease, though this might only relate to antibody being present within the cells. The difference of susceptibility of coeliac mucosa to soluble mediators shown in Falchuk's experiments comes to mind. Could it be that the same or related genes code for both an abnormal immune response to gluten and an abnormal behaviour of the jejunal mucosa? Or could the abnormalities found in the mucosa merely be an expression of the immune response within it?

To cease speculating and conclude, the weight of evidence strongly suggests that an abnormality of the immune response, genetically controlled, is an important factor in coeliac disease. Which particular aspect of the immune response is responsible for the lesion is not clear; sensitised cells or antibodies, or both, may be involved.

Malabsorption and Infection of the Gut in Immunodeficiency

Failure of function of the immune system can be either a congenital or an acquired defect, and of either T cells or antibodies, or both. Congenital deficiency of antibody production causes surprisingly little gastrointestinal disease, except for the occasional association of selective IgA deficiency with coeliac disease mentioned previously. A congenital defect in T cells, however, usually causes diarrhoea and malabsorption, the mucosa shows damage to the epithelial cells and an infiltrate of lipid filled macrophages. Colonisation of the gut by Candida albicans often exacerbates the disease.

Adults can develop an acquired hypogammaglobulinaemic immuno-deficiency that causes malabsorption in about a third of instances. This deficiency is frequently complicated by intestinal Giardia lamblia infection. There is villous atrophy similar to that in coeliac disease, but there is no mucosal plasma cell infiltrate. Occasionally nodular hyperplasia of the gut lymphoid tissue develops. Partial improvement of symptoms follows treatment of any Giardia lamblia infection and some, but not all, patients respond to a gluten free diet.

Pernicious Anaemia

Pernicious anaemia resulting from atrophic gastritis is a condition where, as in coeliac disease, immune attack on mucosal cells causes a failure of absorption, but in this case specifically of vitamin B_{12}. The deficiency follows immune destruction of the parietal cells of the gastric glands, and formation of autoantibody to their product, 'intrinsic factor'. This protein is secreted into the gut lumen, where it combines with the vitamin, and aids its absorption and transport across the ileal mucosa. As the vitamin is an essential coenzyme for DNA synthesis, lack of it interferes with cell division in haemopoiesis, causing the characteristic anaemia.

There is little doubt that the pathogenesis of atrophic gastritis is an autoimmune attack on the parietal cells. Auto-antibodies are present in the serum in 80-90 per cent of cases, and can be demonstrated by indirect immunofluorescence. These antibodies also occur in apparently healthy people, with a frequency increasing sharply with age, but gastric biopsy in these cases invariably shows some degree of atrophic gastritis, giving rise to a concept of *latent* pernicious anaemia. Both the manifest and latent forms of pernicious anaemia are associated with autoimmune thyroid disease, where the gland is destroyed in an analogous manner, with juvenile diabetes mellitus and Addison's disease.

Antibodies to intrinsic factor are present in the serum in 50-70 per cent of cases, and are also found in the gastric juice. There are two types of antibody. Type I inhibits the combination of B_{12} with intrinsic factor, and is common; Type II combines with intrinsic factor, but allows its reaction with B_{12} to take place. It is much rarer. They may be significant in removing small but otherwise adequate amounts of intrinsic factor produced by a depleted gastric-parietal cell population.

The strong association of auto-antibodies with the disease is not proof of guilt. Cell mediated immunity to intrinsic factor has been demonstrated by lymphocyte transformation and lymphokine production. Atrophic gastritis and pernicious anaemia occur in association with hypogammaglobulinaemia (low levels of gamma globulin in the circulation), where, not surprisingly, no serum auto-antibodies can be detected. In these patients, however, lymphocyte sensitivity to intrinsic factor is still present. The lesions in all cases can probably be attributed to cell mediated immunity, rather than the autoantibodies, a finding similar to that in other autoimmune diseases.

Future Developments

Research on relationships of nutrition and immunology began in the nineteenth century and was active in the 1920s, when it produced papers still important today. The more recent voluminous literature has led to our quite extensive insight into topics that are of considerable medical importance. How will understanding grow in the future? Perhaps there are some leads ahead and gaps to be filled that can be extrapolated from the present state of the art.

Absorption of undigested, immunologically active, dietary protein is essential for immune stimulation by the diet. Quantitative data on absorption are sparse in normal subjects, and non-existent in disease. Theories on the aetiology of dietary allergy hinge on the levels of absorption. More information is required and adequate techniques, e.g. radioimmunoassay, now exist.

The level of immune response to dietary antigens is controlled by tolerance inducing mechanisms, by suppressor T lymphocyte activity, by liver function, and possibly by IgA antibody. Suppressor T cells are also involved in controlling the formation of IgE antibodies that lead to dietary and other allergies. Advances in the understanding of these factors will be important in alimentary immunology.

Circulating immune complexes are probably responsible for the distant complications of ulcerative colitis, Crohn's disease and coeliac disease, and may be derived from dietary or gut bacterial antigens. Determination of the nature of the antigens in the complexes will reveal their origin. One study suggested that rabbit atherosclerosis could be exacerbated by immune complexes produced by the feeding of soya bean meal. Further results are awaited with interest, and may have implications for the widespread use of soya bean in human nutrition.

Further studies on T lymphocytes are required to elucidate the complexities of the effects of protein malnutrition on the immune system of experimental animals. The hypothesis was proposed in section 4 that T lymphocyte subpopulations are differently affected at certain levels of protein deprivation, to explain the discordant effects on cytotoxicity and cooperation with antibody forming cells. This should be testable in the mouse.

The failure of the inflammatory response in human malnutrition is probably an important factor leading to infection, but its exact cause is not known and should be explored. The relative importance of protein/calorie against other forms of malnutrition in damaging the immune response in man is not certain. Animal experiments suggest that deficiency in pyridoxine or lipotrophic factors have a severe inhibitory effect. Attention should be paid to these factors in man; if treatment with them were effective in restoring the immune response, it could prove valuable to the management of malnutrition.

Notes

1. R.M. Suskind (ed.), *Malnutrition and the Immune Response,* Kroc Foundation Series, vol. 7 (Raven Press, 1977).
2. I.e. where the colon has been diverted to open on to the skin of the abdomen.

References and Further Reading

Bleumink, E., 'Food Allergy. The chemical nature of the substances eliciting symptoms', *World Review of Nutrition and Dietetics,* vol. 12, 1970, p. 505.
Davis, J.A. and Dobbing, J. (eds.), *Scientific Foundation of Paediatrics,* Heinemann Med., 1974.
Ferguson, Anne and MacSween, R.N.M. (eds.), *Immunological Aspects of the Liver and Gastrointestinal Tract,* MTP Press, 1976.
Goldstein, G.B. and Heiner, D.C., 'Clinical and immunological prospectives in food sensitivity. A review', *J. Allergy,* vol. 46, 1970, p. 270.
Poston, R.N. and Davies, D.F., 'Immunity and Inflammation in the Pathogenesis of Atherosclerosis', *Atherosclerosis,* vol. 19, 1974, p. 353.
Roitt, I.M., *Essential Immunology,* 3rd edn., Blackwell, 1977.
Strober, W. Falchuk, Z.M. *et al.* 'Pathogenesis of Gluten Sensitive Enteropathy', *Annals of Internal Medicine,* vol. 83, 1975, p. 242.
Symposium on Nutrition and Immunology. Proceedings of the Nutrition Society, 35, 253, 1976.
Thomas, H.C. and Parrott, D.R.V. 'Induction of Tolerance to a Soluble Protein Antigen by Oral Administration', *Immunology,* vol. 27, 1974, p. 631.
Walker, W.A. and Isselbacher, K.J., 'Uptake and Transport of Macromolecules by

the Intestine. Possible role in clinical disorders', *Gastroenterology*, vol. 67, 1967, p. 531.

Walker, W.A. and Isselbacher, K.J., 'Intestinal Antibodies', *New England Journal of Medicine*, vol. 297, 1977, p. 767.

Wright, R. (ed.) 'Immunology of GI and liver disease', *Clinics in Gastroenterology* vol. 5, no. 2, 1976.

NOTES ON CONTRIBUTORS

G.J. Ebrahim is Senior Lecturer in Tropical Child Health at the Institute of Child Health, London.

R.J. Jarrett is Senior Lecturer in Epidemiology in the Department of Community Medicine, Guy's Hospital Medical School and Honorary Consultant at Guy's Hospital, London.

R.N. Poston is a Lecturer in the Department of Immunology at Guy's Hospital, London.

INDEX